A Disease
Called
Childhood

AVERY • a member of Penguin Group (USA) • New York

A Disease Called Childhood

WHY ADHD BECAME AN
AMERICAN EPIDEMIC

Marilyn Wedge, PhD

Published by the Penguin Group
Penguin Group (USA) LLC
375 Hudson Street
New York, New York 10014

USA • Canada • UK • Ireland • Australia
New Zealand • India • South Africa • China

penguin.com
A Penguin Random House Company

Most Avery books are available at special quantity discounts for bulk purchase for sales promotions, premiums, fund-raising, and educational needs. Special books or book excerpts also can be created to fit specific needs. For details, write Special .Markets@us.penguingroup.com.

Library of Congress Cataloging-in-Publication Data

Wedge, Marilyn.
 A disease called childhood : why ADHD became an American epidemic / Marilyn Wedge, PhD
  p.   cm.
 Includes bibliographical references and index.
 ISBN: 978-1-58333-563-5
 1. Attention-deficit hyperactivity disorder—United States.   2. Attention-deficit hyperactivity disorder—Social aspects—United States.   3. Child rearing—United States.   I. Title.
  RJ506.H9W432   2015   2014045248
  618.92'8589—dc23

Printed in the United States of America
10 9 8 7 6 5 4 3 2 1

Book design by Lauren Kolm

For Jess, Dan, and Jay, with love

CONTENTS

• • • • • • • • •

A Season in Childhood

In 1988, when I started my practice as a child therapist, I had barely heard of attention-deficit/hyperactivity disorder, or what is typically called ADHD. The diagnosis had arrived on the scene a year earlier, in the third revised edition of the *Diagnostic and Statistical Manual of Mental Disorders (DSM-III-R)*, the book doctors use to diagnose mental disorders in children and adults. Previous iterations of the manual had identified various types of hyperactivity and attention problems in children, including attention deficit disorder (ADD), the precursor to ADHD, in 1980. But this was the first time the term ADHD as we know it today appeared. According to the *DSM*, to warrant a diagnosis of ADHD, a child had to exhibit eight symptoms of hyperactivity, inattentiveness, or impulsivity (from a checklist of fourteen) for at least six months. The checklist included things such as "is easily distracted" or "often interrupts" or "intrudes on others."

Despite its codification in the *DSM*, at the time ADHD was not widely discussed among child therapists, let alone parents, teachers, and pediatricians, as it is today. Psychoanalytically minded child therapists (those inspired by the work of Sigmund Freud) saw children's problems as the expression of inner conflicts, while family systems therapists like me considered kids' problems responses to stressful situations in their social context: at home, at school, or with their friends. We saw no reason to formalize a diagnosis for behavior that child therapists had been successfully treating for years. So we ignored it.

For a while, that was fine. From the time I started my practice until the middle of the 1990s, not one mother or father ever asked me if I thought their child had ADD or ADHD. If their child's behavior changed, parents assumed something was worrying or stressing their child. They came to me to discover the source of stress.

From my point of view, behavioral problems such as aggression, disobedience, or other behaviors commonly associated with ADHD, such as inattention and hyperactivity, are signs that something is wrong in a child's life—either extreme trauma, like abuse or poverty, or something more typical, like a lack of discipline or a difficult family transition. Children are not fully developed mentally or behaviorally. Negative emotions that arise from lack of structure or difficult circumstances in their environments usually manifest themselves in their behavior, since children are not equipped to express themselves directly. I was used to treating children's symptoms as responses to rough patches in their family life or troubled relationships with friends or at school. I helped children cope with sadness or anxiety, compulsive behaviors or aggressiveness, inattentiveness at school or moodiness at home by discovering the cause of the child's distress.

Of course, I saw plenty of children who were jumpy, disruptive, fidgety, oppositional, or uninterested in school. In these cases, parents generally came to me to ask if I could help them keep the behavior in check, sometimes after a teacher had complained that a child was interrupting class or refusing to do assignments. I typically came up with behavioral solutions for these kids. I advised parents to create a solid plan for discipline, to stay calm, not to yell, to give their child time to mature, to reward good behavior, to invoke consequences for mischief, and so forth. At times, I attended a meeting at the child's school and worked with the child's parents, teacher, and school counselor to find specific ways to help the child in the classroom. For particularly active kids—more often boys than girls—I recommended that parents enroll them in a sport or encourage them to ride their bikes as an outlet for their extra energy. Even in cases where something specific—such as divorce, a parent's injury or illness, or another disruption in the child's life—was causing the distress, I could usually work with parents and children to address the problem, talk to the child, and figure out a way for them to move past it. These techniques usually worked.

Not every misbehavior was rooted in a troubling situation at home. In those days, some degree of naughtiness and wildness was tolerated and even expected in children, especially in boys. If parents had a little Dennis the Menace at home, well, that was just boys being boys. Impulsive, distractible kids who occasionally rebelled against the authority of adults were considered naughty but normal. Nobody would have suggested that Dennis the Menace or Beaver Cleaver had a mental disorder that required medication. Nobody would have suggested that Huck Finn's chronic truancy was the sign of a mental illness. A teaspoon of discipline, not a dose of psychiatric medication, was the cure for naughty children. Most people thought the only "disease" that afflicted kids like that was called childhood.

Toward the end of the 1990s, I began to see changes in my practice. More children were coming in to be evaluated for ADHD, often on the recommendation of their teachers. Around 2000, a worried father brought his six-year-old son, Liam, to see me after the boy's teacher said he wasn't keeping up with the rest of his class. The teacher worried that even though Liam was bright, he was falling behind. Liam's father was an epidemiologist with a medical degree from UCLA. He told me in a grim voice that he thought his son had ADHD. I was struck by the fact that he seemed to think of ADHD as a disease that needed to be treated—something you *have* rather than a series of symptoms you exhibit. But I couldn't blame him. The number of children who were being diagnosed with ADHD was skyrocketing. By 2000, approximately 7 percent of children in the United States had the diagnosis, up from 3 percent in 1987. By 2014, the number was 11 percent for children and 15 percent for high school kids. It did seem like an epidemic.

Liam wasn't fidgety or squirmy, but he had trouble focusing and finishing his schoolwork. Sometimes he'd forget to bring home his backpack and would miss several homework assignments. I discovered that Liam was one of the youngest children in his first-grade class. Some of his classmates were already seven, whereas Liam had turned six just before he started first grade. Perhaps, I thought, he simply lacked the maturity to keep up with his classmates in the fast-paced, academically oriented elementary school he attended.

I recommended that Liam's mother and father take turns sitting down with him in the evening while he did his homework and offer him help when he needed it. I suggested they keep the television turned off during homework time so that the noise wouldn't distract him. The parents also made an arrangement with Liam's teacher to contact her by e-mail if Liam forgot to bring home his backpack. The teacher would then e-mail them the homework assignment for that day so Liam wouldn't fall behind. With the extra support and attention, Liam soon caught up with the other students.

Fortunately, we were able to resolve Liam's school problems without referring him to a doctor for medication. However, the epidemic continued to grow for many children. By 2010, Centers for Disease Control and Prevention data indicated that more than ten million American children and teens had been diagnosed with ADHD in doctors' offices. Medication became the go-to solution for kids who were hard to control or struggled at school. Doctors typically prescribed psychostimulant medications such as Ritalin and Adderall to help kids sit still and focus. These medications were not new in the medical arsenal— stimulants had been used to treat nasal congestion, obesity, and mild depression since the 1930s, but they had been newly positioned for children. By 2012, almost twenty-one million prescriptions for Ritalin and Adderall were being dispensed for children each year, up from fewer than three million prescriptions in 1990.

The drugs also became the catalyst for a radical change in the culture of American parenting. Parents came to believe that in an increasingly competitive world, children could no longer afford to dawdle or daydream and learn at their own pace. Kids who didn't apply themselves to their academics were jeopardizing their futures. The media barraged parents, teachers, and doctors with the message that the gap between young people with college degrees and those without degrees was getting wider. From the moment a child entered school at four or five years old, each day mattered.

Kids needed to prepare earlier and earlier for higher education and the workforce. If medication could help them finish high school and get into a good college, parents believed it was their responsibility to medicate their children. The Great Recession of the early twenty-first century exacerbated these trends and accelerated the acceptance of ADHD medications. Childhood itself was getting a makeover, becoming a race to the top instead of a romp on the playground.

There's no question that this attitude was well intentioned. Parents want their kids to have good lives as adults. In a shrinking job market and an increasingly competitive society, parents saw education as the key to their children's long-term success and happiness. They came to believe that stimulants were the answer if their child was struggling because they could help him focus better in school. And as the number of kids taking these medications continued to increase, it became more normal. Like doping in professional sports, you needed a performance enhancer if you wanted to compete.

Unlike many of my therapist colleagues during the first decade of the twenty-first century, as the number of stimulant prescriptions for children rose, I did not refer children to physicians for ADHD medications. I don't think any child without actual neurological damage from disease or injury needs to take a psychiatric medication, whether Ritalin or Adderall for ADHD, antidepressants such as Zoloft or Lexapro, or the dozens of others on the market. Medications can of course manage symptoms and even sculpt a child's personality into a form that is more pleasing and acceptable to adults. But I believe psychiatric medications only conceal, rather than treat, the real cause of a child's troubles. I am not opposed to psychiatric medication for adults. Many anxious and depressed adults believe it has helped them, and it can offer the most seriously disturbed among us the chance to lead normal lives. However, when psychiatric medications are prescribed to most adults, it is best that it be for the short term and accompanied by psychotherapy. When it comes to children, however, I have seen no indication, either in my research or in my own clinical experience, that the diagnoses or medicinal treatments that work for adults apply to kids.

By 2011, many of the children who came to my office were already taking psychiatric medications, prescribed by child psychiatrists or pediatricians. Some of them were so heavily dosed with two or three psychotropic drugs that they seemed more like sedated zombies than active children. I decided it was time to put a stop to the disturbing "quick fix" response to children's problems by the psychiatric community. These children were suffering and the causes of their suffering were not being addressed—indeed, they were being concealed.

In response, I wrote a book called *Pills Are Not for Preschoolers: A Drug-Free Approach for Troubled Kids* to offer parents ways of helping children's emotional problems without medication. I applied family therapy techniques to a wide variety of childhood troubles: anxiety, depression, suicidal thoughts, and compulsive behaviors, as well as behavior and school problems. The book was well received. Soon I was getting e-mails from parents all over the world asking me to help them find a family therapist. One especially moving e-mail came from a father who had returned from deployment in Iraq to find his ten-year-old son taking ADHD medication. He knew his feisty son was a handful and his wife was doing the best she could to help him do well at school. With a little research and a lot of e-mailing back and forth, I helped this father find a family therapist near his town. Six months later, he wrote to tell me that his son was doing well at school and no longer needed medication. Parents from as far away as India and Chile wrote to me asking why their children were prescribed medication for misbehaving at school. What was ADHD, these parents wanted to know, and were there alternatives to medication?

As I watched the ADHD epidemic grow I began to wonder if children in other parts of the world had ADHD in the same numbers as in the United States. In 2012 I happened to read *Bringing Up Bébé*, a charming book about child rearing in France. I couldn't help but notice that the author, Pamela Druckerman, did not mention ADHD. Were French kids somehow escaping the epidemic? What about children in Finland or England? I decided to find out.

My research on ADHD in Europe led me to write an article on my *Psychology Today* blog called "Why French Kids Don't Have ADHD." In writing this, I was inspired by the work of medical sociologist Manuel Vallée, who wrote a cross-cultural study of ADHD in the United States and France. In my article, I argued that French child psychiatrists and neurologists view ADHD differently from their American counterparts. In the United States, child psychiatrists consider ADHD to be a biological disorder with biological causes, and the preferred treatment, psychostimulant medication, is also biological. French child psychiatrists, on the other hand, believe that ADHD is psychosocial and situational. Instead of treating children's focusing and behavioral problems with drugs, French doctors prefer to search out the underlying issue causing a child distress—not in the child's brain but in the child's social context. They then treat the social context problem with psychotherapy or family counseling.

The response to "Why French Kids Don't Have ADHD" was overwhelming. The article attracted national and international attention. It received more than seven million hits, making it the most widely read and shared article in the history of *Psychology Today*. Readers translated the article into French, Norwegian, Portuguese, Greek, Spanish, and a host of other languages. Parents, doctors, therapists, and educators who read the article felt moved to contact me. Many people, especially Europeans, expressed support for my point of view. They were shocked at the idea that so many American children were diagnosed and medicated. They speculated that overcrowded classrooms, lack of physical exercise, the hectic pace of life, and even America's reliance on highly processed foods made our kids hyperactive. Some Europeans were concerned that the ADHD epidemic would spread to their own countries. A neuroscientist from Lyon, France, Dr. Bruno Harlé, told me that French child psychiatrists were feeling strong marketing pressure from drug companies to diagnose ADHD and prescribe medication.

Not surprisingly, American parents were divided in their reactions to the article. Some parents disagreed with me and insisted that ADHD was a neurological condition with similar prevalence in all countries and that stimulant medications had transformed their children's lives. Other parents told me how they helped their ADHD-diagnosed children with nonmedical interventions. "Witnessing the changes in my own son in only one week of eliminating artificial colors from his diet, no one can tell me that diet change doesn't work," wrote one mother from Ohio. A school nurse from Pennsylvania told me she was "sad" to see so many children at her school taking ADHD medications without the social context causes of their problems being addressed. A mother from Massachusetts who gave her son medication after he was diagnosed with ADHD wrote: "My son is finishing college and doing well. He took himself off the medicine during middle school saying he didn't like it." One California mother said that although her son had symptoms of ADHD at school, when she removed him from the school and homeschooled him, his symptoms disappeared. A mother in Germany told me that when a doctor diagnosed her daughter with ADHD and prescribed medication, "we bought her a piano instead—with terrific results."

This dramatic response to my article indicated that I had hit a nerve. There was a pressing need for more information, understanding, and awareness about ADHD. Parents were looking for answers. Was ADHD a true illness that required medication? Were these medications safe for children over the long term? What about making changes in a child's diet or giving children outlets for their energy and creativity? Were the ADHD diagnosis and the drugs used to treat it overturning our society's conception of childhood? And should we as a society be doing better for our kids? These are the questions that inspired me to write *A Disease Called Childhood*.

Why should you listen to me? I have been a practicing family therapist for twenty-five years, specializing in problems of childhood and adolescence. Through my work and research, I have come to understand the ADHD diagnosis and why it has become so ubiquitous in America in a way that I think most parents and practitioners of child and family therapy will find beneficial.

Based on my research, as well as my clinical experience with thousands of children and families, I believe ADHD is a constellation of symptoms that our society interprets as a medical condition for reasons that will become clear in this book. ADHD certainly "exists," in the sense that many children exhibit behaviors that parents and teachers can see and doctors can measure. But in my view ADHD is neither an unnatural condition of childhood nor an illness that requires medication. Often, behaviors tagged as ADHD are normal childhood responses to stressful situations. I believe ADHD is overdiagnosed and overmedicated and that well-meaning parents from all backgrounds have been duped into believing that their perfectly normal and healthy child needs powerful psychostimulant medications just to be "normal" and successful. I believe this is harmful to parents and to children, and I believe there is a better way.

I also believe that American culture is in no small part to blame for the spread of the ADHD diagnosis. Not all cultures, even advanced industrial cultures, see illnesses and their treatments in the same way. What we view as normal or abnormal behavior depends on the mainstream beliefs or norms of the society in which we live.

Therefore, not only medicine, but also culture and society, must enter into our understanding of the ADHD epidemic. I started to explore this in my article "Why French Kids Don't Have ADHD," but I aim to go even deeper in this book. If ADHD were really a disease or disorder that could be treated—like Alzheimer's, say—one would expect the rates of diagnoses to be similar in societies that are genetically similar to ours—namely Westernized and European cultures. But this is not the case. In America, children from all socioeconomic and ethnic backgrounds have been prescribed medication for ADHD, whereas in many European countries, both the diagnosis and medication are used much less. Why is this so?

In this book I share my experience and my findings about the many surprising factors that play a role in ADHD. I tackle the research on a genetic link for ADHD as well as brain imaging techniques that purport to depict ADHD in the brain. I evaluate the studies on dietary interventions for ADHD symptoms, and I especially look at how American culture has allowed the diagnosis and drug treatment to spread like wildfire through our children.

I hope this book will reassure parents that although their child's symptoms certainly are real, and parents have every right to be concerned, there is nothing medically wrong with a child who has been diagnosed with ADHD, except in extreme cases. Let me be perfectly clear: I have written this book not to blame well-intentioned parents for choosing to medicate their children but to help and inform them. Parents have the right to know that there is a wide variety of nonmedical solutions for helping inattentive and overactive children. These include making changes in a child's diet, finding the educational environment that suits the child, understanding the effects of media on children, parent coaching, and family therapy. I will explore all of these in this book. My hope is that the book will spark a reevaluation of the disorder that has led to the wholesale drugging of America's children and the medicalization of American childhood.

PART I

An
American
Epidemic

ONE

What Is ADHD?

> If a man does not keep pace with his
> companions, perhaps it is because he
> hears a different drummer.
>
> • HENRY DAVID THOREAU

I met Aiden in 2008 when he was seven years old. The previous year, he had moved with his family from New York to California, and the transition had been difficult. He missed his friends in his old neighborhood and his cousins who had lived nearby. When I met with Aiden's parents, Scott and Ava, they told me Aiden had always been a handful. Even as a baby Aiden was colicky and fussy, and difficult to put down to sleep. At two years old, he was more active than most of their friends' children. Aiden's preschool teachers had been concerned about his disruptive, impulsive behavior.

Now Aiden's second-grade teacher said he typically fidgeted at his desk and talked with his classmates instead of completing his class work. Often he doodled or daydreamed and missed the teacher's instructions so the teacher had to explain an assignment two or three times before he figured out what he was supposed to do. The teacher sent notes home almost every day. Worst of all, Ava explained with tears in her eyes, Aiden was beginning to feel bad about himself. He had begun saying things like "I hate myself" and "I'm stupid."

On the plus side, Ava told me, Aiden was a sweet and caring child. He seemed to be able to focus for hours on things that interested him such as video games. He was also an amazing artist. The walls of their house were covered with his drawings of horses, their cat Donovan, and their dog Barney. He had been playing piano since he was five, and his piano teacher said he had a natural talent for music.

Worried about Aiden's disruptive behavior at school, Ava and Scott took him to the pediatrician. The doctor said Aiden had enough symptoms of hyperactivity, impulsiveness, and inattention to warrant a diagnosis of ADHD.

At the time, the current edition of the *DSM* was the *DSM-IV*, which had expanded the definition of ADHD from that in the *DSM-III-R* into two categories: a) inattentive and b) hyperactive/impulsive. The manual then defined three subtypes of ADHD: 1) ADHD, Primarily Inattentive; 2) ADHD, Primarily Hyperactive/Impulsive; and 3) ADHD, Combined Type.

For a diagnosis of the primarily inattentive ADHD, a child must have six or more symptoms of inattention, without having six symptoms of hyperactivity or impulsivity. The manual outlined these symptoms as follows:

INATTENTION

1 • Often fails to give close attention to details or makes careless mistakes in schoolwork, work or other activities
2 • Often has difficulty sustaining attention in tasks or play activities
3 • Often does not seem to listen when spoken to directly

4 • Often does not follow through on instructions and fails to finish schoolwork, chores, or duties in the workplace (not due to oppositional behavior or failure to understand instructions)

5 • Often has difficulty organizing tasks and activities

6 • Often avoids, dislikes, or is reluctant to engage in tasks that require sustained mental effort (such as schoolwork or homework)

7 • Often loses things necessary for tasks or activities (e.g., toys, school assignments, pencils, books, or tools)

8 • Is often easily distracted by extraneous stimuli

9 • Is often forgetful in daily activities

For a diagnosis of ADHD, primarily hyperactive/impulsive, the child must have six symptoms of hyperactivity and/or impulsivity without having six symptoms of inattention. These included:

HYPERACTIVITY

1 • Often fidgets with hands or feet or squirms in seat

2 • Often leaves seat in classroom

3 • Often runs or climbs excessively in inappropriate situations

4 • Often has difficulty playing quietly

5 • Is often "on the go" or acts as if "driven by a motor"

6 • Often talks excessively

IMPULSIVITY

7 • Often blurts out answers before questions have been completed

8 • Often has difficulty waiting for a turn

9 • Often interrupts or intrudes on others

For the combined type, a child must have six symptoms of inattention and hyperactivity. For a diagnosis of any of the three types, the child's symptoms had to last for at least six months, with some impairment in at least two settings (e.g., home and school). Some symptoms had to be present before the age of seven.

Aiden had been diagnosed with the combined type because his behaviors fit the criteria for both hyperactivity/impulsivity and inattention. The pediatrician wrote a prescription for Adderall. Before giving Aiden the medicine, however, his parents decided to consult me to find out if there was some other way to help him apart from medication. I was happy to help.

A Brief History of ADHD

To fully understand how ADHD is diagnosed and why there are so many different versions of it, a little historical background is in order. I mentioned in the introduction that ADHD was first introduced in 1987 with the publication of the *DSM-III-R*, but similar collections of symptoms had gone by a series of different names and definitions over time.

The first appearance of hyperactive behavior in a psychiatric manual was in the *DSM-II*, published in 1968. The diagnosis "hyperkinetic reaction to childhood," according to the American Psychiatric Association, which authors the manual, was characterized by "short attention span, restlessness, distractibility and overactivity, especially in young children." The authors added that this type of immature behavior in children "usually diminishes in adolescence."

The *DSM-II* also listed another childhood diagnosis that was characterized by symptoms similar to hyperkinetic reaction to childhood but had a different cause. They called this disorder mild brain damage or "organic brain syndrome." Doctors had observed that children stricken with encephalitis, which injured their brains, exhibited symptoms that were nearly identical to the symptoms of hyperkinetic reaction to childhood. Many children had contracted encephalitis during the epidemic of 1918–1930, with resulting damage to their brains. These children appeared restless, impulsive, overactive, and easily distractible, and they were diagnosed with mild brain damage.

Though the symptomatic behaviors of hyperkinetic reaction to childhood and mild brain damage were nearly identical, the authors of the *DSM-II* gave them different names to reflect their different causes. The cause of hyperkinetic reaction to childhood was psychosocial, meaning that the symptoms were a reaction to stress in the child's social environment or emotional conflicts within the child. Mild brain damage, on the other hand, was caused by neurological damage from a known brain-impairing disease such as encephalitis, meningitis, or an event of brain trauma. This distinction between behaviors caused by emotional and social factors and those caused by neurological disease or injury is important to keep in mind as we trace the history of ADHD.

In the *DSM-III*, published in 1980, the new diagnosis of "attention deficit disorder" (ADD) replaced hyperkinetic reaction to childhood. According to the new criteria in the *DSM-III*, a child could be diagnosed with ADD if he was distractible, disorganized, had a short attention span, tended to procrastinate, and acted impulsively. These behaviors had to last for at least six months. As we have seen, the term "attention deficit disorder with hyperactivity," or ADHD, made its first appearance seven years later in the *DSM-III-R*. The authors of both versions of the *DSM-III* did not differentiate between attention deficit disorder and minimal brain damage. Instead, they combined the two diagnoses because their symptoms were the same. However, the authors stated that "predisposing factors" for ADHD were central nervous system abnormalities such as those caused by cerebral palsy, epilepsy, and neurological disorders *as well as* "disorganized or chaotic" home environments and child abuse and neglect. By combining two distinct diagnoses into one disorder called ADHD, the authors profoundly changed how mental disorders were defined. Instead of being diagnosed based on *cause*, a disorder was now diagnosed based on *symptoms*. This marked a radical shift in American psychiatry that I will explore more deeply in Chapter 3.

After the publication of the *DSM-III-R*, several studies appeared suggesting that some children could be inattentive and distractible without being hyperactive. To reflect these findings, the definition of ADHD was changed again in the fourth edition of the manual, the *DSM-IV*, published in 1994. The authors of the *DSM-IV* did not change the name ADHD, but they distinguished between inattentive and hyperactive types of ADHD. The *DSM-5* further expanded the ADHD diagnosis by extending the age of onset of the symptoms.

A Creative Child

Aiden's parents, Ava and Scott, had read about the side effects of stimulant drugs such as Adderall, and they were concerned. Aiden was a little underweight and they had read that one side effect of the drug is decreased appetite. More important, they were worried that Adderall might dampen Aiden's creative spirit. Scott was a filmmaker and told me Aiden reminded him of himself at that age. He had been a "hyper" kid, and now he was grateful that his parents had enrolled him in gymnastics and had given him guitar lessons instead of medicating him. Eventually he had grown out of his bouncy behavior.

Scott had read that creative people like Thomas Edison and Albert Einstein didn't do well at school when they were children. He knew that Paul McCartney of the Beatles daydreamed in class and didn't get good grades. McCartney was too busy learning to play the guitar and listening to music to do his homework. Had these creative geniuses been children in today's culture, they might well have been diagnosed with ADHD and medicated. Scott was concerned that a drug that sharpens a child's focus might at the same time curb his ability to think creatively. He was not entirely anti-medication, but both he and Ava had a healthy skepticism about pharmaceuticals.

Scott and Ava asked if I thought Adderall would help Aiden. In the spirit of providing them with all the options, I told them it probably would. Stimulants like Adderall help most children calm down and become more focused. In most cases, the effects of the medication are visible from the first day a child begins taking it. However, if they wanted to go the non-medication route, I told them I was willing to take the journey with them. Aiden wasn't a naughty child. He was just one of those active kids who need to move around in order to think. This kind of child tends to think "outside the box" and isn't especially interested in the typical schoolroom fare of readin', writin', and 'rithmetic. These kids like novelty and challenges. Give them a new video game and they can concentrate for hours.

Moving the Goalposts

Aiden's story is frighteningly common. Since ADHD has become more ubiquitous, more and more parents are turning to professionals when their child starts exhibiting symptoms of inattention or hyperactivity, even if he is otherwise healthy. More often than not, these parents, like Aiden's, walk away with a prescription for Adderall or Ritalin. These are the two drugs most commonly associated with ADHD, but there are a host of others. Doctors can also prescribe Adderall XR (a slow-release version of Adderall), Vyvanse, and Dexedrine, which, like Adderall, are amphetamines, or Focalin and Concerta, which are methylphenidates like Ritalin. While methylphenidate bears some chemical similarity to amphetamine, it is a more complex molecule. Although the two compounds act by different biochemical mechanisms, both lead to an increase in brain neurotransmitters (particularly norepinephrine and dopamine), which accounts for their stimulant activity. Amphetamine (e.g., Adderall) is effective in lower doses than methylphenidate (e.g., Ritalin) but is considered more addictive and is more widely abused. Methylphenidate has different and potentially more significant side effects. There are no clear guidelines on which of these drugs is preferable for any given patient. Decisions by psychiatrists on which drug to prescribe are based largely on personal preference and on simply trying them on the patient.

A liquid form of methylphenidate, Quillivant XR, is available for younger children who have difficulty taking pills. If stimulant drugs don't help, or if the child has an adverse reaction, the next step is a nonstimulant medication such as Strattera or Intuniv. These drugs have different chemical compositions, but they have all proved to be effective in calming children down, correcting unruly behavior, and improving a child's ability to focus on schoolwork. These drugs don't work in every single case, of course, but they have been found to help most children.

As I pause to reflect on children like Aiden and the many others I have seen over the past two and a half decades, I can't help thinking our society has moved the goalposts of normal childhood. What is considered normal behavior for a child is not the same today as it was when I first started seeing children in therapy. One indication of this is that the definitions of ADD or ADHD in various versions of the *DSM* have widened in scope, so that more children are eligible for the diagnosis.

The definition of what is disordered behavior in children and what is normal has shifted—in the eyes of doctors and in the eyes of our society. A child who would not have met the criteria for an ADD diagnosis in 1980 could warrant the diagnosis of ADHD today with the expanded criteria set by the *DSM-IV* and the *DSM-5*. In 1980, a child had to have at least eight symptoms from the checklist to be diagnosed with ADD. A child—let's call him Billy—who had only six symptoms from the checklist did not qualify for the diagnosis. Today, in the *DSM-5*, the number of symptoms has been reduced from eight to six, so today Billy would be diagnosed with ADHD.

And these days the ADHD diagnosis, which started out as a disorder of childhood with symptoms beginning by age seven, has spread to teenagers, college students, and even adults who want to boost their productivity. The *DSM-5* changed the age of onset of symptoms for the ADHD diagnosis. Instead of symptoms beginning by age seven (required in the *DSM-IV*), the diagnosis can now be made if symptoms appear by age twelve. The *DSM-5* also made it easier for a teenager to be diagnosed with ADHD. A teenager need only have five symptoms instead of the six required for younger children.

When you look at how the number of children diagnosed with ADHD has changed as the criteria for the diagnosis have expanded, you can see a definite correlation. In 1970, when the hyperactivity disorders in the *DSM-II* (hyperkinetic reaction to childhood and minimal brain damage) were distinct, only a tiny fraction of American children were diagnosed with symptoms that resemble what we call ADHD today. In 1987, the number of diagnosed children was about 3 percent. By 2003, it was 7.8 percent, in 2007 it was 9.5 percent, in 2011, the latest year for which data is available, it was 11 percent, and by 2014 it was more than 12 percent.

Meanwhile, many children and teens are medicated to enhance their ability to focus on academics, even if they don't strictly qualify for a diagnosis. Many parents I've worked with have reported that Ritalin and Adderall have helped their children focus. There's no doubt that stimulant drugs work to improve attentiveness. The catch is that research has shown that stimulants help *anyone* focus, whether or not they have symptoms of ADHD. Today, 15 to 40 percent of high school students take amphetamines to enhance their focus on tests and boost their grades, and some teenagers and young adults end up in drug rehabilitation programs because they became comfortable with taking amphetamines as children.

With this in mind, I can't help but wonder whether we are actually treating a childhood mental illness with these medications or instead are allowing the drugs to transform our very image of childhood.

A Plan to Help Aiden

When Aiden's parents asked me if I thought Adderall would help their son, I told them it probably would. However, I added that there were other, drug-free ways to get the same results. Scott and Ava decided that even though family therapy might take longer than giving Aiden Adderall, they would give it a try. I helped them come up with a plan for Aiden to get plenty of physical exercise. They enrolled him in tee-ball and began taking family bike rides and hikes on weekends. We explored dietary changes, which sometimes help overactive kids. Ava found that eliminating sugar, gluten, and foods with artificial colors from Aiden's diet had a noticeable effect in calming him down. While not all kids have a sensitivity to these foods, they can be irritating to some children. (We'll talk more about how diet can affect a child's behavior in Chapter 7.) Scott and Ava structured Aiden's time on school days. After school he would have a healthy snack and a glass of milk. He could play outdoors with the neighborhood kids until five, when it was time to begin his homework. After Aiden finished his homework, he would be allowed to play a video game or watch TV for an hour. At bedtime, Scott and Ava took turns reading to him.

Scott and Ava met with Aiden's teacher, school principal, and school psychologist. Together they worked out accommodations to help Aiden. The teacher changed his desk so he sat close to her and away from friends who might distract him. She gave Aiden the responsibility of watering the plants in the classroom and erasing the blackboard. This allowed him to get up and move around as part of his school day. The teacher agreed to make sure Aiden understood the directions for assignments. She would clarify the directions if he didn't understand them the first time. They agreed on a plan for regular home–school communication; the teacher and a parent would sign Aiden's homework so he wouldn't miss assignments.

Over the course of four months, Aiden became much calmer at school. Though he didn't stop daydreaming altogether, with the extra support he became more attentive to his teacher's directions. By the end of the school term, with the increased help at school and at home, Aiden was doing much better. His parents were relieved that he didn't have to take medication.

Medicating Childhood

I applaud Aiden's parents for questioning the effect medication would have on their son. Not only are so many people too quick to medicate hyperactive kids, they have by and large accepted drugs as the preferred treatment of this so-called disorder without considering the side effects. There are medical side effects such as insomnia, decreased appetite, and heart problems, but there are also effects on the child's personality. Recently, a young adult client of mine named Noah told me a story that moved me to reflect on how psychiatric drugs are being used today to reshape personality. Noah, who is twenty-four, came to me after he broke up with his girlfriend. He had read an article I wrote on natural ways to treat depression and was looking for alternatives to medication. When Noah was nineteen, his psychiatrist prescribed the antidepressant Prozac, which did help him become less shy and introverted, but after six months he decided to stop taking it. When I asked him why, he told me he felt Prozac turned him into "a teenage girl." He became overly emotional, crying about the least

little thing. Unlike many patients whose personalities undergo a welcome transformation when they begin taking Prozac, Noah didn't like
the new personality that came with the drug. He said on Prozac he
didn't feel "like [his] real self." Noah preferred being true to himself, even
shy and depressed, to being the new personality Prozac had sculpted.

Reflecting on Noah's experience, I cannot help but wonder if the
ADHD medications we now give to kids, especially boys (10 percent
of high school boys in the United States currently take ADHD medication), are having an effect on them similar to the effect one Prozac
had on Noah. These drugs enhance a child's ability to focus in the
classroom and help him keep pace in competitive schools and in a
competitive society. But in giving children ADHD drugs are we also re-
shaping their personalities and asking them to give up something
basic to their authentic selves? By nature, young children have a lot of
energy. They are impulsive, physically active, have trouble sitting still,
and don't pay attention for very long. Their natural curiosity leads them
to blurt out questions, oblivious in their excitement to interrupting
others. Yet we expect five- and six-year-old children to sit still and pay
attention in classrooms and contain their curiosity. If they don't, we are
quick to diagnose them with ADHD. In many advanced countries, as we
will see in this book, children are not expected to curb their natural
energies and sit still in classrooms until the age of seven. Not surprisingly, these countries have much lower rates of ADHD. Boys, especially,
are lively and energetic and have more difficulty sitting still than do
girls. On average, boys' brains mature later than girls'. But in the United
States today, we seem to be asking boys to conform to a standard of
behavior that in the past would have been more appropriate for girls.

The notion of mental health or mental illness is relative to the values of a particular society at a particular time in history. Our hectic society paradoxically frowns on overly active children—even children as young as four or five years old. Our society wants children to be restrained, orderly, and eager to please adults. We have little tolerance for typically boyish traits such as bounciness, fidgetiness, and mischievousness. We want boys to sit still for hours in the classroom without physical exercise, pay attention to their teachers, and not throw spitballs. What's more, as a society we have decided (or at least acquiesced) to drug these annoying traits out of boys. This is more than moving the goal-posts. It is more like changing the game.

Of course this is not the whole story. There are factors other than boyhood that figure into an ADHD diagnosis. Girls are diagnosed with ADHD as well, although in fewer numbers. In the United States today, 13.2 percent of boys are diagnosed with ADHD. The percentage for girls is 5.6 percent. In my own practice, girls who have been diagnosed with ADHD and medicated by their doctors are typically "underachieving" at school. They are getting Bs and Cs instead of As, even though they are bright and capable of doing better (though I remember a time when Bs and Cs used to be considered "average," not "underperforming," and parents often rewarded children for getting Bs). Our expectations have changed and parents seek medication for their kids primarily to drive them to raise their grades.

Clearly, some girls are also hyperactive. For them, getting involved in gymnastics or dance can provide a creative outlet for their extra energy. Singer Audra McDonald, for example, disclosed in her 2014 Tony Award acceptance speech that she had been hyperactive as a child. She was grateful that getting involved in theater channeled her energies and saved her from having to take medication. If she had to take medication, would she be the dynamic, creative woman that she turned out to be? What about Aiden? Would Ritalin have taken away his exuberance and his sparkle, which were essential parts of his personality?

There is another aspect of ADHD that worries me. As stimulants have come to be prescribed for ever larger numbers of children, our society's very perception of childhood has changed. Instead of seeing ADHD-type behaviors as part of the spectrum of normal childhood that most kids eventually grow out of, or as responses to bumps or rough patches in a child's life, we cluster these behaviors into a discrete (and chronic) "illness" or "mental health condition" with clearly defined boundaries. And we are led to believe that this "illness" is rooted in the child's genetic makeup and requires treatment with psychiatric medication.

Surprisingly, the likelihood of a child being diagnosed with ADHD in the United States varies according to where the child lives. According to a recent study by the Centers for Disease Control and Prevention, 14 percent of schoolchildren are currently diagnosed with ADHD in Arkansas and Louisiana. In Nevada, the number is less than 5 percent. If ADHD were truly a genetically based biological disease, wouldn't the percentage of children diagnosed with it be more or less equal across geographical areas? Are doctors in Arkansas and Louisiana more skillful at diagnosing ADHD than doctors in Nevada? It seems unlikely.

The Drug Defines the Disease

How did America get to this point? How did our image of childhood evolve so that behaviors once considered normal are now considered a disorder? In his classic book *Listening to Prozac*, psychiatrist Peter

Kramer observed that "psychotherapeutic drugs have the power to remap the mental landscape." Kramer offers the example of the drug lithium. When lithium proved successful at treating symptoms of manic depression, manic depression became ubiquitous. Psychiatrists, he says, have always longed for a model in which one particular drug would fit one specific disease. In *Prozac Nation*, Elizabeth Wurtzel also discusses the one drug/one disease phenomenon. She says that her doctors defined her illness as "depression" because she responded to a specific antidepressant drug, Prozac. The drug defined her disease.

Like Kramer, Wurtzel also noticed that a psychiatric drug not only came to define a particular mental disorder, but the drug also expanded that disorder across society. She observed, too, that the process was driven by profits to drug companies. The discovery of a new drug to treat depression resulted in many more patients being diagnosed with depression. She watched this occur through the 1990s, as Prozac and a number of other new antidepressants arrived on the market. As new antidepressants became available, the diagnosis of depression expanded until it medicalized almost every aspect of human sadness—from premenstrual blues to the natural grief people feel following the death of a loved one.

I think Wurtzel's and Kramer's observations about how a psychiatric drug can both define and expand a psychiatric diagnosis were prophetic. The same thing that occurred with Prozac and depression, and with lithium and manic depression, is occurring today with stimulant medications and ADHD. The response to stimulant drugs has both defined and expanded the scope of the ADHD diagnosis. Stimulant medications have changed the societal landscape such that today ADHD has become a household word. Ten million American children have received the diagnosis in our country, and the epidemic is spreading abroad. ADHD is the diagnosis du jour, just as depression was the favored diagnosis in the 1990s. Of course, the new "illness" is perceived as biological because it has a convenient biological treatment.

As Wurtzel points out, the process of defining a disease by a drug is illogical and backward. Medicine has traditionally defined diseases by their causes, not by the drugs to which patients with similar symptoms respond. If psychiatry aspires to be scientific, on a par with other branches of medicine, how can it be content with this peculiar practice of delineating the outlines of a disease by a drug treatment? Can you imagine if other diseases were treated this way—if a person was diagnosed with high blood pressure because medication reduced his blood pressure? In the next chapter we will see that not every society has redefined the norms of childhood (and especially boyhood) in such a way that a large percentage of its children are diagnosed with a "mental disorder" called ADHD. Not every society has embraced mental steroids to enhance their children's academic performance and control their behavior. They have found other ways to deal with the often annoying juiced-up energy level of childhood.

TWO A Tale of Many Cultures

We believe that classifying these problems as "illnesses" misses the relational context of problems and the undeniable social causation of many such problems.

• BRITISH PSYCHOLOGICAL SOCIETY

While I was researching and writing "Why French Kids Don't Have ADHD," I made the surprising discovery that illnesses and their treatments, especially in the field of mental health, are not as universal and objective as we might think. What is considered a mental illness and what is not is shaped in large measure by cultural values and traditions. What doctors regard as a disease in one country can change when a patient crosses a border and enters a country with an equally advanced system of medicine. So it is with American psychiatry's peculiar notion that ADHD is a neurobiological illness and that dosing overactive or inattentive children with stimulants is an acceptable—and even preferred—treatment. Whereas children all over the world exhibit inattentive, impulsive, and hyperactive behaviors, not all cultures view these behaviors through a medical lens. Stimulant medication for children has become socially acceptable in the United States, but this is not the case in all advanced countries and has not always been so in the United States.

One sign of the variability in the social acceptance of stimulants is that the United States consumes 70 percent of the world's stimulant drugs, though it represents only 4 percent of the world's population. Other countries with first-rate medical systems have different perspectives on the childhood behaviors that American psychiatry classifies as ADHD. A child in the United States is six times more likely to be medicated for ADHD than a child in France and sixty times more likely than a child in Finland.

Thanks to our acceptance of pharmaceutical drugs and the murky classification system of the *DSM*, which we discussed in the previous chapter, American child psychiatrists view children's difficult behaviors as a neurodevelopmental condition with a biological cause. But in countries like France, Finland, and Italy, doctors have a somewhat different perspective. The difference stems in part from their own medical traditions and in part from a vigorous skepticism of the research that purports a biological cause for ADHD.

Childhood behaviors that signify a medical condition to American doctors are more likely to signify a problem in the child's social environment to a French one. A French child psychiatrist typically views ADHD-type behaviors as signaling not a deficiency in the child's brain chemistry but rather a malaise in the child's life. Perhaps the child's parents are experiencing stress. Perhaps the child is having problems with friends or is having difficulty keeping up at school. A French psychiatrist would more likely recommend family therapy, individual therapy, and/or school interventions than stimulant medication for a child's problems.

The French holistic, psychosocial approach also allows for considering nutritional causes for ADHD-type symptoms—specifically the fact that the behavior of some children is worsened after eating foods with artificial colors, certain preservatives, and/or allergens. Medication would only be a last resort and would not be the sole treatment. When stimulants are prescribed, they would be accompanied by psychotherapy and/or school interventions. While the number of children in France taking psychostimulants has increased in the past ten years—about 1 percent of school-age children take the drugs, according to a recent Pharma-funded telephone survey of parents—that number is still significantly lower than in the United States, where the percentage of children medicated with stimulants is 6 percent.

In Finland, stimulant medication is prescribed for only one in one thousand children, a mere 0.1 percent of the child population. Finns view inattentive and hyperactive behaviors as an educational challenge that typically would be addressed by a team of professionals at the child's school. In Finland, the question of whether or not a child needs additional educational support is based not on a medical diagnosis but on a teacher's observations of the individual child's needs. We will explore the Finnish approach to education and childhood in Chapter 6. Italy's attitude toward diagnosing and medicating children for ADHD-type behaviors is similar to the French and Finnish views. Hyperactive or inattentive behaviors signify a problem in the child's family, social, or educational environment, and the typical solution would be family therapy and/or school interventions.

France Resists the *DSM-III*

When the *DSM-III*, with its new biological conception of ADD, arrived in France in 1980, French child psychiatrists responded with a firm *Arrêtez* (Stop)! French child psychiatrists even wrote their own manual of childhood mental disorders as an alternative to the *DSM-III*. As you recall from the last chapter, the *DSM-III* was the first manual to combine the two different types of hyperactivity instead of distinguishing them by their causes. All of a sudden, two diagnoses—one caused by environmental or developmental factors, the other caused by brain damage from a disease or head injury—were considered one and the same. According to the *DSM-III*, children with documented neurological damage and normal children who were going through a developmental phase were classified in the same way. Therefore, at least according to the *DSM*, these children should be treated the same way as well.

These ideas alarmed French child psychiatrists because they differed so radically from the French diagnostic process. When the cause of a child's problem was not an organic factor such as brain damage from disease or injury, French psychiatrists looked for a social environment cause. They considered the whole child in his social context—his family life, his personal history, his experiences at school, and his relationships with friends. Abstracting a troubled child from his lived context and reducing him to a checklist of symptoms was at odds with the French tradition of psychiatry and French child psychiatry's developmental approach to mental disorders.

The Reforms of Pinel

To get a deeper understanding of French psychiatry, we must take a brief look at history. At the end of the eighteenth century, two great reformers—Philippe Pinel in France and William Tuke in England—humanized the treatment of the mentally ill, who up to that time had been treated little better than animals. Since I am discussing the French tradition, I will focus on Pinel. Famous for "liberating the insane from their chains," Pinel directed reforms at the Bicêtre Asylum and later at the Salpêtrière Hospital in Paris. Reading the recommendations in medical texts led Pinel to wonder, in a surprisingly modern vein, "whether the patient or his physician has the best claim to the appellation of a madman." He distrusted the so-called scientific beliefs of his era regarding organic causes and "pharmaceutic" cures of madness. Instead, Pinel emphasized careful observation of patients, including monitoring how seasonal and weather changes affected their moods and behavior. Through daily conversations with his patients, he learned how their symptoms emerged from their life experiences. He discovered that the financial ruin and personal losses that many patients had suffered during the French Revolution brought out madness in people who had previously led perfectly normal lives.

In *Treatise on Insanity*, Pinel offered case descriptions so clear and detailed that his patients come to life before our eyes. He listened with great interest to their stories about their disappointments in love and their failures in business. He also devised ingenious strategies to fit his patients' individual situations. For example, one of Pinel's patients, a farmer, had suddenly become insane for no apparent reason. Talking with him, Pinel discovered the farmer's sons had committed him to the asylum in order to take possession of his home and his land. He understood right away that such a betrayal by one's children was enough to drive a father insane. Pinel arranged with the local magistrate to have the sons evicted and the ownership of the farm restored to the father. After this, the farmer regained his sanity, moved back to his house, and resumed his productive life without suffering a relapse.

Thus began a long tradition in France of considering a patient's history and social environment in mental disturbances. The same is true today for children's problem behaviors. French child psychiatrists had long believed that severe cases of childhood hyperactivity and impulsivity, when not accompanied by an obvious biological cause for the symptoms, were rooted in emotional distress or psychological conflicts arising in the child's life experiences. French child psychiatrists also recognized that many hyperkinetic and attentional problems were developmental phases that children often grow out of without any kind of intervention. These kids might be annoying or difficult to teach, but immaturity was the cause, not a biological disease.

Kraepelin's Classification of Mental Disorders

Long before American psychiatry published the *DSM-III*, the French had resisted a similar type of classification of mental disorders. As the profession of psychiatry grew through the 1800s, European doctors became concerned with creating a common language for understanding mental diseases. They wanted a way to communicate with each other about their patients, especially patients with serious mental illnesses. In 1883, a gifted German psychiatrist named Emil Kraepelin attempted to classify all the known mental disorders in a small book. Through the years, Kraepelin went on to identify over a hundred diagnoses, which eventually filled a larger book called *Psychiatrie*. Psychiatrists and neurologists in most European countries accepted Kraepelin's impressive classification system. But French psychiatrists weren't buying it. They criticized Kraepelin for being nonsystematic and for lacking a theoretical basis for his classifications.

French psychiatrists had their own views on classification. In 1860, the psychiatrist Bénédict Morel described dementia praecox, or *démence précoce*, as a type of dementia or chronic mental confusion that afflicted young people. However, Morel also believed that environmental factors—such as local climate and customs, housing conditions, work, diet, and alcohol—influenced some forms of madness. Pierre Pichot, a modern French psychiatrist and past president of the International Psychiatric Association, has remarked, "The adherence by the French school to its original principles of classification makes it difficult to translate French diagnoses into other systems." In the next century, this recalcitrance to accept foreign classifications of mental disorders was to serve France—and especially French children—well.

In response to the *DSM-III*, the French Federation of Psychiatry produced its own manual of child psychiatry, the *French Classification for Child and Adolescent Mental Disorders* (*CFTMEA*), which was published in 1983 and was updated in later editions. Written by a task force led by child psychiatrist and professor Roger Misès, the *CFTMEA* was created with one goal in mind: "to offer French psychiatrists an alternative to the *DSM-III*." According to Misès and his team, "French child psychiatrists worried that *DSM-III* was quite different from the clinical process that most of them were using for diagnosis decision making. They also worried that the *DSM-III* could drastically change clinical practices by focusing all of the clinical and therapeutic attention on isolated symptoms."

The *CFTMEA* was validated through a broad study that included professionals from most child psychiatric facilities in France and was used by child psychiatrists with various theoretical orientations. Unlike the *DSM-III*, it maintained a distinction based on causes. Causes were divided into organic factors (e.g., genetic mental retardation or brain injury) and environmental factors. Hyperkinetic and attentional disorders were recognized under the environmental category. The *CFTMEA* focused on identifying and addressing the underlying psychosocial causes of children's symptoms, not on managing the symptoms with pharmacological balms. The French manual also outlined narrower criteria than the *DSM-III* for diagnosing hyperactivity and attention problems, thus reducing the number of children eligible for the labels. For example, the *CFTMEA* explicitly discourages giving a child a diagnosis of hyperkinesis if the child has attention problems but not hyperactive behavior. The *DSM*, as we have seen, allows a diagnosis of ADHD (inattentive type) even when the child shows no signs of hyperactivity.

Jacques Lacan and France's Psychoanalytic Tradition

Besides adopting a different manual, there were other reasons France resisted the onslaught of biological child psychiatry. Unlike in the United States, where psychoanalysis had been defeated by biological psychiatry (a subject we'll discuss further in Chapter 3), psychoanalysis was a strong presence in France when the *DSM-III* landed on its shores. Prior to 1960, French psychiatry had rejected psychoanalysis for being too pragmatic and focusing too much on problem solving; but in the late 1960s, psychoanalysis in France was transformed and rejuvenated, thanks to the influence of the seminal psychoanalyst and philosopher Jacques Lacan. Lacan, sometimes called the "French Freud," infused psychoanalysis with creative new ideas that made it more humanistic and appealing. According to Massachusetts Institute of Technology sociologist Sherry Turkle, Lacan's ideas inspired France to become a "psychoanalytic culture." Psychoanalytic metaphors and ways of thinking entered into not only the world of intellectuals but also into the language of everyday life. Lacan had a call-in radio show that was one of the most popular shows in the history of French broadcasting.

Nonetheless, when antidepressants became available in the 1980s and 1990s, French adults availed themselves of the drugs even more than Americans. In his 2012 book, *Psychotropic Drugs: The Investigation*, reporter Guy Hugnet found that more than one in five French adults took antidepressants. But, unlike Americans, the French did not succumb to the allure of stimulant drugs for their children. The French government refused to relax the prohibition on direct-to-consumer advertising of pharmaceutical drugs. French parents were therefore spared magazine ads for Adderall XR that pictured a smiling mother hugging her smiling child holding a paper with a B+ on it. As we will see, American parents and children were not as well protected from such marketing.

Against this historical backdrop, a fierce ideological battle between the two traditions of psychiatry is playing out on the world stage today. One side (the neo-Kraepelinian biological psychiatrists) holds that ADHD symptoms constitute a distinct biological disorder, even without brain damage from recognized diseases or brain injury. The other side (the psychoanalysts, humanists, social psychologists, and family thera-pists) maintains that ADHD is simply a catchall name for social, emo-tional, and developmental issues of childhood.

While attitudes vary from country to country, there is a strong back-lash against American biological psychiatry's view of children. Euro-pean parents, teachers, and doctors have resisted using medication to treat ordinary childhood behavior problems and are looking for alter-natives. Family and school interventions, such as consistent discipline and more physical exercise and play during the school day, are consid-ered appropriate treatments for hyperactivity, impulsivity, and atten-tional problems. As we saw in the previous chapter, these are the same types of things I recommended to Aiden's parents in lieu of Adderall.

Even though more than thirty years have passed since the publi-cation of the *DSM-III*, European countries still prefer to use the World Health Organization's *ICD-10* (*International Classification of Diseases 10*, shortened title of the *International Statistical Classification of Diseases and Related Health Problems*) instead of the *DSM-5*. The *ICD-10* criteria for hyperkinesis are narrower than the criteria for ADHD in the *DSM-5*, and fewer children qualify for the diagnosis. The *ICD-10*, like the *CFTMEA*, requires a child to display hyperactivity as well as inattention, with onset before age six, for a diagnosis of hyperkinetic disorder to be made. The diagnostic process for children also differs from that in the United States. In France, in order to evaluate a child for a diagnosis of ADHD, a child psychiatrist, pediatrician, or pediatric neurologist care-fully interviews the child and the family for at least eight sessions. Stim-ulants are not prescribed for children under the age of six. In Italy, the diagnosis must be made by a pediatric specialist.

In the United States, by contrast, the diagnostic process is much more casual. Not only child psychiatrists and pediatricians, but also family practitioners, internists, and nurse-practitioners are allowed to diagnose ADHD and prescribe stimulant medications for children, sometimes based on no more than a twenty-minute evaluation using a checklist of symptoms. American regulations concerning psychiatric drugs for children, which are less rigorous than those in many European countries, also make it possible for American doctors to prescribe stimulants to children much more frequently than their European peers.

It is worth pausing to note that German psychiatry was much more accepting of the *DSM-III*. Even today, German psychiatrists tend to see ADHD as a chronic biological disorder, best treated with medication. The prevalence of the disorder in Germany is higher than in France, at 4.8 percent of children (as of 2008, the most recent date for which data are available). In Germany today, the use of stimulants for children diagnosed with ADHD is among the highest in Europe, although still significantly lower than in the United States.

Looking at how other cultures view childhood issues adds depth and nuance to the over-medicalized American approach. A major 1984 study in Italy shines a light on the ways in which different cultural traditions influence how doctors view childhood problems. The same clinical case information was presented to an American and an Italian team of psychiatrists and pediatricians for assessment. The clinical information included symptoms and behaviors typical of a child with ADHD. The teams came up with two different conclusions. The American team interpreted the issues within an organic and biological framework, whereas the Italians interpreted the same case information with a psychodynamic and socio-environmental perspective. The Americans diagnosed "hyperactivity" or "behavioral disorder," while the Italians chose to view the problems as "personality disorder" and "learning disability."

Although there is a heated national debate in Italy between groups who advocate "the right to Ritalin" versus those who support "the right to childhood," the number of Italian children diagnosed and medicated for ADHD-type symptoms, at 1 to 2 percent, is far lower than in the United States. Italian culture is loath to accept the widespread drugging of children. The Italian ministry of health tightly controls stimulant prescription, and a parent cannot simply purchase Ritalin at a pharmacy. Only pediatric specialists at authorized centers can prescribe ADHD medications, and the prescriptions are filled on-site. Italy does not allow pharmaceutical companies to infiltrate schools by handing out "educational materials" to parents. While Italian doctors recognize the characteristics of ADHD as deviant and unusual, most of them do not think of ADHD as a biological syndrome or a distinct diagnostic entity. Instead, they consider ADHD-type symptoms to be on a continuum with normal childhood behaviors.

Parenting

Another way in which culture shapes a child's behavior involves parenting. Again, we can look to France for a dramatic alternative to American parenting. Several recent books praise the benefits of French parenting, especially with respect to discipline. Despite the books' fanciful titles, like *French Children Don't Throw Food* (the American title is *Bringing Up Bébé*), they offer serious wisdom. It is worthwhile, then, to take a closer look at how French parents manage to raise children to be well behaved and focused, while, by all accounts, they are as loving and attentive as their American counterparts.

French parents share the conviction that children need a structured environment for their emotional health. Structure and predictability, the French believe, make a child feel safe and secure. From the time their children are born, French parents provide them with a firm *cadre*, which means "frame" or "structure."

French parents are strict about a few key things—bedtime, the amount of television their kids can watch, and mealtimes. Mealtimes are at four specific times of day, and French children learn to wait patiently for meals and are not allowed to eat unhealthy snacks whenever they feel like it. And meal times do not revolve around children's soccer schedules or their favorite television programs. In France, meals are about "sitting at the table with others, taking one's time and not doing other things at the same time," say French sociologists Claude Fischler and Estelle Masson. Within the basic *cadre*, French parents give their children appropriate choices. For example, a child may not be allowed to eat sweets between meals, but at the traditional afternoon snack time around 4 p.m. (the *goûter*), they can eat small helpings of cookies, chocolate, or cake. When I lived with a French family during a brief stay in Paris, I always looked forward to strawberries with cream at the *goûter*.

The French believe that clear limits actually make a child feel happier and safer. Giving a child love without limits and discipline, writes Pamela Druckerman in her popular book *Bébé Day by Day*, produces a little tyrant—or what the French call an *enfant roi* (a child king). The battle cry of French parents is "It's I who make the decisions." Their kids are granted choices, but not total freedom. Children are expected to behave well in the presence of adults, including at mealtimes. Psychologist Tiffany Field, of the University of Miami School of Medicine, studied French and American preschool children. She found that French three-year-olds behave admirably in restaurants. They eat their meals quietly and do not argue, throw food, or refuse to eat, as many American children do. She also observed that French preschool children on playgrounds were less aggressive to their playmates than are American preschoolers. As both a therapist and a parent, I can attest to the power of consistent structure and parental expectations in getting children to behave appropriately.

Pamela Druckerman observes, in *Bringing Up Bébé*, that French parents believe hearing the word "no" rescues children from the "tyranny of their own desires." French children do not fall apart when they don't get their way. They have learned that a tantrum, however loud or embarrassing to the parent, will not change a no to a yes. As a mother who often pushed a shopping cart up the aisle with three young children in tow, I understand that saying no and sticking to it is not easy. But French parents know that if they are consistent in not rewarding misbehavior, children will understand that throwing a fit is futile.

French children don't need medications to control their behavior because they learn self-control early in their lives. They grow up in families with a clear hierarchy and established rules. In French families, parents are firmly in charge of their kids, in contrast to the American family style, in which the situation is all too often reversed, with the entire household centered on the children. Our egalitarian culture has encouraged us to be friends to our children rather than authority figures, and we hesitate to say no for fear of losing that friendship. American parents like their kids to have a say in the rules that concern them, whereas French parents have no qualms about making the rules themselves. And French parents manage to have affectionate relationships with their children despite, or perhaps because of, the clear unspoken hierarchy of authority in French families. I am not implying that French parents are inherently better than American parents. This is not at all what I mean. I am simply pointing out that French culture preserves traditional attitudes and conventions about childrearing that support parents in setting clear boundaries and that these boundaries affect the way a child behaves.

A psychosocial view of ADHD-type symptoms suggests that a child's family interactions can influence the emergence of behavioral and attentional problems. This correlation between how children are raised and how they behave is not lost on child development experts. Thus, research in Europe and the United States is focusing on the role parenting plays in ADHD symptoms. A major Swedish study in 2010, conducted by researchers at Stockholm University and the Karolinska Institutet, looked at more than one million children, ages six to nineteen. The researchers found that family factors such as parents' lack of time to spend with children, financial problems in the family, lack of social support, and family conflict, including separation and divorce, can all correlate with a child being diagnosed with ADHD.

Substantial research indicates that teaching parents certain types of skills can provide the same benefits as prescribing pills. Parenting experts in the United States and other countries are developing education programs to teach mothers and fathers healthy parenting skills, especially appropriate discipline techniques. These programs are based on research indicating that inconsistent, overly harsh, or overly permissive child rearing can result in behavior and attention problems in children. One such program is called "The Incredible Years." In Ireland, for example, a four-year evaluation by an international research team concluded that the Incredible Years training effectively reduced ADHD-type symptoms in children without the use of medication. Researchers found that children whose parents attended a twenty-week training made significant progress in reducing their hyperactivity and inattentiveness. The children also displayed increased social skills several months after their parents had completed the program.

The Incredible Years and similar programs emphasize the effectiveness of calm consistent limit setting without using harsh measures such as spanking or yelling. Programs like this reflect a growing awareness that the parenting environment can affect children's behavior and attentiveness, and may in some cases be a substitute for ADHD medication. The Incredible Years and other programs have spread to Norway, Portugal, Spain, New Zealand, and a host of other countries. On our own shores, a program at the Center for Children and Families at the State University of New York at Buffalo has had good results. In a study involving 128 families with a child diagnosed with ADHD, psychologists found that one third of the parents who completed the program saw enough improvement in their children that they decided that drugs were unnecessary. The other two thirds put their children on stimulant drugs on school days only, but at significantly lower doses than typically prescribed.

The fact that parent coaching can reduce the incidence and severity of hyperactive behavior casts real doubt on the belief that ADHD is a biological disorder; it also suggests that making changes in the way we parent could protect our children from developing ADHD in the first place. Parenting active children certainly presents a special challenge that requires particular skills. One American father, after completing an education program for parents of ADHD kids in upstate New York, compared parenting his unruly son to driving a Mack truck. Everyone can learn pretty quickly to drive a car, the father said, but to drive a Mack truck people need some extra training. After he and his wife participated in a parent training program, where they learned how to discipline their son consistently and calmly, the boy was able to get back on track at school without taking medication.

Many of the ingredients of the parent education programs complement the intuitive attitude French parents seem to have about discipline. The rules of the *cadre* make overly harsh or overly permissive discipline unnecessary. French parents also insist on having a life and identity of their own apart from the kids, something parents in the training programs found to be a great stress reliever. And French early childhood education, which does not put academic pressure on young children, may even deter ADHD.

In French public preschools, which children can attend until they turn six, children are not taught to read. Though some kids pick up reading earlier, French children are not formally taught to read until first grade, when they turn seven. This attitude reflects the teachings of Swiss psychologist Jean Piaget, who believed that children reach educational milestones at their own pace. Trying to speed them up from their natural pace doesn't make any sense to his conception of child development. To the north of France, the small country of Finland has a similarly relaxed attitude about early education. In Finland, children start school during the year they turn seven. Forcing kids to sit in classrooms before this age is considered a violation of the rights of children to be children. In the California suburb where I live, if a child is not read-ing by the age of six—or preferably even earlier—her concerned par-ents send her to an after-school learning center to boost her skills or seek a diagnosis of ADHD and medication. Taking a long view at other cultures reveals this as our own cultural bias. I take a closer look at cul-tural differences in children's education in Chapter 6.

Despite a growing number of alternative ways of viewing and treat-ing children who struggle at school, diagnosing children with ADHD and medicating them with drugs is still the mainstream point of view of American psychiatry. In the next two chapters, 3 and 4, I discuss how the ADHD epidemic gathered steam in the United States through a confluence of potent social and economic forces: influential academic child psychiatrists, insurance companies, the "me" generation of par-ents, and—above all—the pharmaceutical industry.

PART II

· · · · · · · · · · · · · · · · · · ·

How Did
We Get
Here?

THREE

How a Diagnosis Became an Epidemic

> Make a habit of two things: to help or at
> least to do no harm.
>
> • HIPPOCRATES

As this book unfolds, you will understand why the ADHD epidemic in the United States is raging at full force with no signs of slowing down. As we have seen, the *DSM-5* significantly broadens the diagnosis, ensuring that the epidemic will sweep even more children and teens into its grasp than ever before. We have seen that one reason many European countries have not experienced the same rates of ADHD as the United States is their reluctance to embrace the *DSM*'s style of categorization. Certainly the cultures and laws of countries such as France, Italy, and Finland have played a role in keeping the ADHD epidemic at bay; but when one studies the history of this new form of psychiatry, it's clear just how vital it's been in America's willingness to medicalize behavior.

As I explained in the previous chapters, one central principle of the new model of psychiatry was the view that children's attentional problems were a discrete mental disorder caused by a hypothetical defect in the child's brain. Implicit in the new psychiatry was a de-emphasis on social, emotional, and environmental factors as possible causes of children's psychological and behavioral problems. The new psychiatry created a framework of classification and checklists, with a narrative of neurotransmitters and chemical imbalances, and of observable behaviors—all of which removed children from the rich and complex tapestry of their lived experience. To understand what a profound shift this was in American psychiatry, it's useful to have some background.

Individual and Environment

The ancient Greek physician Hippocrates of Cos, often credited as the father of medicine, taught that in treating illness a doctor must look at the patient's social and physical environment—including his diet, geography, and living habits—along with the patient's physical symptoms. For Hippocrates, individual human beings were products of their natural environments. The dualistic thinking that separated living beings from their habitats had not yet been introduced in Western medicine and Western culture. But this artificial disconnection between human beings and their environment is as critical in leading our thinking astray as the more famous mind-body dualism usually blamed on the French philosopher René Descartes. Thinking about a living being as detached from an environment is as abstract and misleading as thinking of our minds as separate from our bodies.

Gregory Bateson, an ecologist and an early pioneer of family therapy, famously said, "The unit of survival is the organism *and* its environment." Emotional health depends in large part on being in an environment—both social and geographical—that feels natural for us. When a polar bear at the Winnipeg Zoo began constantly pacing back and forth, she was diagnosed with depression and given Prozac. It is obvious that the bear was not suffering from a biological disorder but rather from an unnatural and unhealthy habitat. The social and physical environments in which we live and work have a direct influence on whether we—humans and polar bears alike—feel well or ill, happy or discontent. Abnormal and even diagnosable behaviors, like the pacing of the polar bear, could be seen as an adaptation to an unhealthy situation rather than as an illness best treated by a drug.

For children, parents are the most important environmental influence on their well-being. And children are much more exquisitely attuned to their parents' feelings and their relationship with them than most parents probably realize. Teachers, too, are important influences on a child. Every parent knows that having a teacher who is not a good match can make a child irritable, anxious, or inattentive.

DSM-I and DSM-II

Before the emergence of what is now known as "biological psychiatry"—the notion that behavioral and mental disorders are caused by biological factors rather than environmental ones—and its embodiment in the *DSM-III*, psychiatrists took the patient's environment into account. Childhood problems were viewed as reactions to stress in the child's social environment or as developmental hurdles. Earlier editions of the diagnostic manual, the *DSM-I* and *DSM-II* (issued in 1952 and 1968, respectively) reflected a concern with the underlying environmental causes of childhood troubles. Diagnoses were described as "reactions" to stressors in the child's world. Thus, a child's diagnosis was not set in stone as a *quality* of the child or as a permanent medical condition. Rather, children's symptoms were viewed as fluid and subject to change with proper interventions or simply with maturity. Ordinary language reflected this point of view. For example, we used to say that a child was "going through a phase" to explain an "abnormal," odd, or uncharacteristic behavior.

The doctors who authored the *DSM-I* and *DSM-II* were trained in psychoanalysis, the dominant theory in American psychiatry at that time. The philosophy of the first and second editions of the diagnostic manual presented a psychodynamic approach to human problems. This paradigm, based on Freud's research, focused on internal conflicts arising from early childhood trauma. Freud's experience with hysteria and other maladies of the mind had led him to conclude that psychological distress was a reaction to a dysfunctional or abusive social environment in childhood. Freud was particularly concerned with emotional trauma, an extreme form of stress. He believed that traumatic events in early childhood were "the source of the Nile (*Caput Nili*)" of all serious emotional problems. These problems were subject to change through treatment with talk therapy, known famously as Freud's "talking cure."

Authors of the *DSM-I* and *DSM-II* maintained this understanding. Young children could be rowdy and teenagers typically felt anxiety. These could be treated with family interventions and/or child psychotherapy, or simply by waiting until the child matured out of the developmental phase.

Psychiatry in Upheaval

In the 1970s, American psychiatry was becoming more fragmented and diverse. There were multiple constituencies in the American Psychiatric Association, each with its own ideas about the etiology (causes) of psychological problems and treatment. Moreover, the profession of psychiatry itself had been weakened by a frontal attack by the antipsychiatry movement, defined by influential thinkers such as R. D. Laing, Thomas Szasz, and Michel Foucault, who criticized psychiatry for medicalizing the unconventional. Laing believed mental illness was a normal reaction to a dysfunctional family or a dysfunctional society. Szasz believed that psychiatry should be concerned with human relationships, not with medicating individuals. Foucault emphasized the traditional importance of the doctor-patient relationship for healing human troubles, a relationship that disappeared when psychiatry narrowed its focus to diagnosis and classification.

Another group criticized psychiatry for being unscientific. Psychiatric diagnoses were widely known to be unreliable. In 1949, the psychologist Philip Ash had published a study showing that three psychiatrists, when faced with the same patient, reached the same diagnosis only 20 percent of the time. Another researcher, psychiatrist Aaron Beck, found that psychiatrists agreed on a diagnosis between 32 and 42 percent of the time. These numbers made diagnostic labeling seem little more than random and subjective. How could doctors hope to find a cure for a patient when they didn't know what condition they were treating? The low-reliability issue led to a loss of government research funding to the field, which was a blow to psychiatry's claim to be medical science. Between 1963 and 1972, the number of grants that the National Institute of Mental Health (NIMH) awarded to psychiatry declined by 16 percent. Third-party payers had also become skeptical of psychiatry as a legitimate field of medicine. Psychiatric problems seemed like a bottomless pit for insurance companies. They wanted to pay for "real diseases," not for upsetting life situations, and began to restrict the number of sessions of psychiatric treatment for which they would pay.

Finally, the introduction of new psychiatric medications in the 1950s and 1960s, such as chlorpromazine (Thorazine) for schizophrenia and lithium carbonate (Lithobid) for manic depression fueled a heady optimism that biological solutions would become available for all psychological problems. Weakened by the antipsychiatry movement's challenges to their credibility, the loss of funding, and the success of new psychiatric drugs, psychoanalysis was on the verge of being dethroned by a new theory of psychiatry that would claim to be more objective and "scientific."

This new model originated in the work of three psychiatrists at Washington University at St. Louis in the 1960s and 1970s: Eli Robins, Samuel Guze, and George Winokur. The "Wash. U. trio" (as they later became known) were dissatisfied with the current state of American psychiatry. They theorized that faulty biology, not psychological conflicts, caused human troubles. Diseases of the mind, they believed, were essentially the same as diseases of the body. As in other branches of medicine, the goal of the psychiatrist should be to find a specific biological (i.e., drug) treatment to correct a specific biological deficit.

In 1966, a talented resident named John Feighner arrived at Washington University to study biological psychiatry with Robins, Guze, and Winokur. Feighner believed that ideally each psychiatric diagnosis would have one specific treatment. A correct diagnosis would point the doctor to the right drug cure. However, in the state of psychiatry in the 1960s and 1970s, this was not always the case. Patients with the same diagnosis did not always respond to the same treatment. It became painfully clear to Feighner that the state of psychiatric diagnosis was a mess. As an example, he described two patients diagnosed with schizophrenia who responded differently to the same treatment. One of the patients responded poorly to electroconvulsive therapy (ECT) but positively to antipsychotic drugs. The other responded positively to ECT but poorly to antipsychotics. The diagnosis of schizophrenia, therefore, could scarcely be correct in both cases. Feighner believed psychiatry needed to refine diagnostic criteria so as to be able to pinpoint specific disorders.

Feighner went on to develop diagnostic criteria for psychiatric disorders. Robins, Guze, and Winokur were coauthors of the paper and the diagnostic criteria became known as the "Feighner criteria." The criteria were lists of symptoms for twelve disorders, without reference to any underlying causes of the patient's distress. The goal of psychiatry, as Feighner and the Wash. U. trio saw it, was to classify symptoms into a specific diagnosis, abandoning any attempt to identify the underlying social-context causes of a patient's troubles or to acknowledge the importance of the relationship between doctor and patient. According to the Wash. U. group's way of thinking, underlying psychosocial causes were too tied up with psychoanalytic theory to be of use, and the therapeutic benefit of the doctor-patient relationship could not be measured and was therefore unscientific. The psychiatrist's role, as Feighner saw it, was to classify and diagnose, not to enter into a moral relationship with the patient.

The Allure of Classification

Psychoanalytic theory had put forth a spectrum view of human troubles. For Freud and later psychoanalytic therapists, there was no sharp boundary between the mentally normal and the mentally sick. Given unhappy circumstances such as disappointment in love, death of a loved one, or financial ruin, any human being could become severely depressed or even have psychotic symptoms. The new biological model, however, held that there was a sharp boundary between mental illness and mental health. A person was either sick or well. Biological psychiatrists therefore took issue with the *DSM-II*, which had been influenced by psychoanalytic theories.

Robins, Winokur, and Guze dreamed of changing American psychiatry and they succeeded. In the words of a contemporary psychoanalyst, they caused "an upheaval in American psychiatry which will not soon be put down." Two historical developments helped them along the way. First, the introduction of new psychotropic drugs presented unbounded research possibilities. Second, in 1971 Robins met New York psychiatrist Robert Spitzer, who would later be appointed chairman of the *DSM-III*. As a result of their influence on Spitzer, the Washington University group would transform psychiatric practice from the art of healing into the medical-pharmacological behemoth we have today. Naturally, one side effect of a biological model was that the preferred treatment was biological as well, a notion that the pharmaceutical companies that produced psychotropic drugs quickly embraced. We'll look more closely at the role Big Pharma had to play in the spread of ADHD in Chapter 4.

Robert Spitzer and the *DSM-III*

Robert Spitzer graduated from the New York University School of Medicine in 1957 and practiced psychiatry at the Columbia University Center for Psychoanalytic Training and Research. He became dissatisfied with psychoanalysis because he felt it didn't help his patients improve. In 2005, the *New Yorker* published an article looking back on the making of the *DSM-III* and quoted Spitzer expressing his frustration with psychoanalysis: "I don't think I was uncomfortable with listening and empathizing—I just didn't know what the hell to do." What he did, eventually, was to travel to St. Louis to "sit at the feet" of Eli Robins (in the words of Spitzer's colleague Paula Clayton). In 1975, Spitzer and Robins wrote a paper that elaborated on the Feighner criteria, and Spitzer later included the criteria in the *DSM-III*, along with nine additional criteria that he and Robins devised.

When Spitzer was appointed head of the *DSM-III* task force, the job was of little importance. Most psychiatrists in the APA didn't expect much to change with the new revision and therefore didn't take much interest in it. Columbia University psychiatrist Donald Klein remarked that one of the reasons Spitzer got the job was that it wasn't considered that important. Previous versions of the *DSM* were of interest to only a small select audience. Nor were the APA trustees aware when they appointed Spitzer that he already had in mind specific plans for the new *DSM*. Spitzer intended to resolve the reliability problem by nailing down detailed criteria for each mental disorder. To this end, he filled the *DSM-III* committees with psychiatrists influenced by the Wash. U. biological approach.

The *DSM-III* and the biological model set the course for the future of American psychiatry. Spitzer scarcely could have envisioned the dramatic and far-reaching impact of his manual in shaping American culture and society. The *New Yorker* article captured that impact in a few well-chosen words: "[Spitzer] not only revolutionized the practice of psychiatry but also gave people all over the United States a new language with which to interpret their daily experiences and tame the anarchy of their emotional lives." Through the biological lens of the *DSM-III*, psychiatrists reduced the complexity of human problems to discrete "medical" conditions, which they believed functioned under objective, unchanging rules. The biological psychiatrists also had a significant advantage over other psychiatric orientations. They were to enjoy unprecedented financial backing from pharmaceutical companies, which were all too happy to fund their research on the efficacy of drug treatments.

Classification is no doubt enticing. Distinguishing one thing from another and giving things names is a basic human instinct, giving order and meaning to the confusion of individual experience. However, classification of symptoms without reference to their causes is not itself a science. This sort of classification does not help the doctor decide on a cure. For example, a sore throat, stuffy nose, and cough could be caused by either a viral or a bacterial infection. The treatment depends on the cause of the symptoms. For a bacterial infection, the doctor may prescribe an antibiotic. For a viral infection, the doctor would offer medicines for symptomatic relief but not an antibiotic. The classification of respiratory infections into bacterial and viral is scientific because it refers to the causes of the symptoms. The presence of a bacterial infection can be determined by a laboratory test if necessary.

Decades after the *DSM-III* was published, when the hypothesized biological causes of the disorders in the manual still eluded psychiatry, despite billions of dollars poured into research by drug companies, Spitzer came to regret the whole enterprise of biological psychiatry. By then, however, the damage had been done.

The Drug Pipeline

By the late 1970s—the years in which the *DSM-III* was being written and readied for publication—pharmaceutical companies had become powerful forces within the medical community. They provided substantial funding for psychiatric researchers and contributed to the funding of the American Psychiatric Association's conventions. And of course they reaped substantial profits from the expanding markets for psychiatric medications. Pfizer, one of the country's largest drug companies, funded the development of a method called PRIME-MD (Primary Care Evaluation of Mental Disorders). PRIME-MD allowed doctors to use checklists to make a psychiatric diagnosis in an average of eight minutes. Pfizer would of course stand to benefit if more doctors prescribed its antidepressant Zoloft, which it introduced in 1991.

In the 1990s, Pfizer financed symposia to train six thousand primary care physicians in the use of PRIME-MD. Spitzer, who was one of the main developers of PRIME-MD, was thus responsible for greatly expanding the number of doctors who were able to diagnose mental disorders and prescribe psychiatric medications. Now family practitioners and internists could diagnose and treat mental disorders after a short, intensive training, even though they had little or no training in psychiatry or psychology. As *DSM-III* critics would later note, PRIME-MD became the "Alaska pipeline" for pharmaceutical companies, facilitating their direct access to a lucrative new market.

With the publication of the *DSM-III*, arriving at a correct diagnosis and finding an effective drug to suppress symptoms became the focus of therapy. In the new biological psychiatry, diagnosis became focused on counting up behavioral symptoms and classifying them into a disorder. ADHD, for example, was classified as a "disruptive behavior disorder." Doctors merely had to go through a checklist of observable behaviors, find a diagnosis for the patient, and prescribe the appropriate drug.

This meant child psychiatrists no longer felt the need to listen at length to the subjective narratives of parents and children. The new biological psychiatrists no longer believed a therapist's interaction with a patient could help a patient on its own. The therapist became a simple observer, a classifier, rather than a healer. Freud's "talking cure," which was based on a dynamic, interactional model of therapy, was replaced by a doctor who matched a patient's symptoms with a disorder and prescribed drugs. Biological psychiatry had indeed created an Alaska pipeline not only to adults, but to millions of children as well. In the decades to come, that pipeline would become immensely profitable for America's drug industry.

With the burgeoning influence of the *DSM-III*, any problems typical of children—not just impulsivity and distractibility, but also irritability, sadness, anxiety, and even naughtiness—were presumed to be biological malfunctions or deficiencies within the child, classified into disorders by symptom checklists. Yet the new biological psychiatry was not without its critics. In 1997, two savvy California professors, Stuart Kirk of UCLA and Herb Kutchins of California State University, Sacramento, criticized the *DSM-III* because it allowed for diagnosing children without considering social context issues such as psychological trauma. Troubled children, they observed, were often victims of "emotional, physical and sexual abuse." They thought it was a serious mistake to pathologize and label children, as this process obscured the real sources of their distress. Kirk and Kutchins were also outraged that "individuals are given *DSM* diagnoses when family, marital, and social interrelationships are clearly the problem."

Voting Is Not Science

In a coup that bore traces of a Freudian revolt against the father, biological psychiatry in America succeeded in overturning its psychoanalytic forebear. The elaborate classification system of the *DSM-III* enhanced psychiatry's scientific aura and prestige and gave it the semblance of being on a par with other branches of medicine. Yet even members of the *DSM-III* task force questioned the manual's foundation in authentic science. Task force member Theodore Millon thought the "science" hadn't really been done. He said there was "little systematic research, and much of the research that existed was really a hodgepodge—scattered, inconsistent and ambiguous. . . . I think the majority of us recognized that the amount of good, solid science upon which we were making our decisions was pretty modest." Diagnoses were included or excluded from the manual not by scientific evidence but merely by taking a vote among the group of authors. Spitzer himself admitted there was little objective research supporting the validity of *DSM-III* disorders. "There are very few disorders whose definition was the result of specific research data," he said. The decision process was more about power politics than about scientific decision-making. "We took over because we had the power," Spitzer later admitted in an interview. Donald Klein, a member of Spitzer's task force, had a similar opinion. "Sure we had very little in the way of data, so we were forced to rely on clinical consensus, which admittedly is a very poor way to do things. But it was better than anything else we had." Ultimately, Klein said, whether or not a disorder was included in the manual was decided by a vote.

The *DSM-III* and the succeeding diagnostic manuals did not solve the reliability issue. The process of diagnosis remains subjective. Even today, one psychiatrist may diagnose a child with ADHD, another may diagnose the same child with bipolar disorder, and a third may give a diagnosis of oppositional defiant disorder. Recently, an eleven-year-old girl arrived at my office diagnosed with all three, for which she was taking three different psychiatric medications. The source of her anxiety, moodiness, and inability to concentrate, I soon learned, was to be found not in her neurochemical makeup but rather in her parents' rancorous divorce.

The ADHD Checklist

The greatest expansion of categories of disorder offered by the *DSM-III* involved children's disorders. As I've mentioned in earlier chapters, the *DSM-III* offered the first description of ADD that combined symptoms of hyperactivity caused by environmental factors and symptoms caused by brain damage under one diagnosis. The diagnosis ADHD appeared on the scene seven years later with the publication of the *DSM-III-R*.

To warrant a diagnosis of ADHD, according to the *DSM-III-R*, a child had to have eight out of the following fourteen symptoms, with typical onset before age four:

1 • Often fidgets or squirms
2 • Has difficulty remaining seated
3 • Is easily distracted
4 • Has difficulty awaiting turn in games or group situations
5 • Often blurts out answers to questions
6 • Has difficulty following through on instructions from others, for example, does not finish chores
7 • Has difficulty sustaining attention in tasks or play activities
8 • Often shifts from one uncompleted activity to another
9 • Has difficulty playing quietly
10 • Often talks excessively
11 • Often interrupts or intrudes on others
12 • Often does not seem to listen to what is being said to him or her
13 • Often loses things necessary for tasks or activities at school or at home
14 • Often engages in physically dangerous activities without considering possible consequences (e.g., runs into street without looking).

Later, with the publication of the *DSM-IV* in 1994, eligibility for an ADHD diagnosis was widened by reducing the number of symptoms required from eight to six, out of a new checklist of eighteen symptoms. New behaviors added to the checklist were:

1 • Often fails to give close attention to details
2 • Often has difficulty organizing tasks and activities

3 • Often avoids, dislikes, or is reluctant to engage in tasks that require sustained mental effort

4 • Often runs about or climbs excessively in situations in which it is inappropriate.

In 1969, a psychologist named C. Keith Conners had created a checklist for parents and teachers to rate a child on symptoms of what was then called hyperkinesis. Conners's list includes many of the behaviors that were in the *DSM*, as well as different categories such as "hard to control at shopping malls or the grocery store" and "only attends if it is something s/he is interested in." Like the *DSM-III*, the Conners rating scale did not consider the underlying causes of the child's behavior. It did not consider the child's life story, apart from symptomatic behavior. Today, the computer-based Conners Continuous Performance Task (Conners CPT) measures children's attention span, impulse control, and response time. A diagnosis of ADHD may be obtained in a mere twenty minutes. The Conners CPT is widely used by psychiatrists and educational psychologists to diagnose hyperactivity.

No Blame

In addition to the influence of pharmaceutical companies and the *DSM-III*, there were other reasons for the success of the biological model. The influence of third parties grew rapidly during the 1970s. Insurance companies required diagnoses for reimbursement and called for a closer relationship between diagnosis and treatment. But an even more significant factor was that the biological model of psychiatry appealed to parents who had often felt blamed when they took their child to a psychoanalytically oriented therapist. Parents became resistant when therapists began suggesting making changes to their parenting model as part of their children's treatment.

In 1978, the child psychoanalyst Dorothy Bloch observed that parents found relief in the idea that their child suffered from a real biological illness, in whose origins they or other family members played no role. Bloch poignantly described her shock and sadness when a mother told her she would prefer to hear that her son was an incurable schizophrenic, rather than consider that changes to her parenting style might improve his behavior. Instead of "blaming" parents for their children's problems, the new biological way of diagnosing children let parents off the hook entirely.

With the coming of the "me" generation and the "culture of narcissism" in the 1970s, the times were ripe for a theory that separated parents' actions from their children's problems. In 1979, psychoanalyst Alice Miller's *The Drama of the Gifted Child* was published to enormous acclaim. The author's chilling stories of the emotional damage narcissistic parents inflict on their children were enough to make even the most well intentioned parent run for cover. Parents did not want to think of themselves as "narcissistic." Although Miller eventually broke her ties with psychoanalysis, in the eyes of the public she was solidly in the camp of parent blamers.

The psychoanalytic theory that maternal coldness (the infamous "refrigerator mother" theory) was the cause of childhood schizophrenia or autism provided a rallying point for parental resistance to the psychoanalytic model. In 1979, the National Alliance for the Mentally Ill (NAMI)—now called the National Alliance on Mental Illness—was founded by two Wisconsin women, Beverly Young and Harriet Shetler.

The women were mothers of sons diagnosed with schizophrenia, and they started NAMI to protest the parent-blaming "refrigerator mother" theory of childhood problems. With the help of drug industry money and the support of the American Psychiatric Association, NAMI quickly gained power as an advocacy organization and stirred the public's negative opinion of psychoanalysis. It was as if the pendulum swung too far in the other direction—the backlash against psychoanalysis wanted to reject any notion that held parents accountable instead of considering that several factors could contribute to a child's behavior. In my own view, children's behavior problems—especially severe problems such as childhood schizophrenia—stem from multiple causes, including the parents' relationship with each other and with their own parents, as well as their relationship with the child. Reducing the cause of serious childhood problems to a "refrigerator mother" seems overly simplistic and unhelpful, but completely rejecting the notion that parents had a role to play in their child's development had its own negative effects.

By 1999, NAMI had received more than $11 million from pharmaceutical companies to reach out to increasingly receptive parents. NAMI used that money to conduct educational programs, meetings, and support groups for parents. It provided a phone crisis line to offer support to parents and youngsters, as well as a magazine and a newsletter that informed families about mental illness and the benefits of psychiatric drugs. The money also helped support their national convention and fund a lobbying group. According to the New York Times, NAMI coordinated some of its lobbying efforts with drug makers and pushed legislation that benefited drug industry products.

Drug industry funding of NAMI continued to grow. The New York Times reported that from 2006 to 2008, drug companies contributed nearly $23 million to NAMI, a whopping 75 percent of NAMI's total donations. NAMI kept its ties to the drug industry secret until it received a letter from Senator Charles Grassley (R-IA) asking about its ties to drug makers. This letter was part of Grassley's investigation of the drug industry's influence on medical practice. In response to Grassley's letter NAMI began listing the names of drug companies that donated $5,000 or more on its Web site.

Eventually, even psychoanalytically oriented child therapists such as Dorothy Bloch and Alice Miller started to reconsider the role that a child's environment, especially parenting, plays in determining the child's emotional health. In her classic book on child therapy, *So the Witch Won't Eat Me*, Bloch was especially adamant on the role of parenting in the etiology of schizophrenia. She wrote, "The continuing reluctance to acknowledge the presence of environmental factors in the genesis of schizophrenia may be traceable to the feelings of guilt and shame that continue to surround the whole area of the parent-child relationship." Bloch inevitably encountered resistance when she tried to work with parents on "repatterning" the way they interacted with their children. Parents usually pulled their children out of therapy at the slightest mention of changing their parenting style, preferring instead to believe that their child suffered from a congenital, incurable illness.

In *The Drama of the Gifted Child*, Alice Miller expressed the view that all mental illnesses are the result of traumas experienced in childhood. Childhood traumas, as Miller conceived them, fell along a spectrum—from outright sexual exploitation of a child by parents to parents denying the child's needs for respect, mirroring, understanding, and sympathy. The specter of psychoanalytic "blame" continued to haunt parents.

Trauma

Another factor that helped fuel the popularity of the biological model was the disillusionment with psychoanalytic therapy. As Spitzer realized in his own practice, psychoanalysis was not useful in resolving the real-life problems patients brought to therapy. Moreover, Freud's views on how early childhood trauma could lead to severe emotional distress later in life were as threatening to twentieth-century American doctors as they were to Freud's tight-laced medical colleagues in nineteenth-century Vienna. In fact, the medical community of Freud's day was so critical of his idea about the connection between childhood trauma and later psychological problems that he felt obliged to retract his views on the subject. This led to his famous revision in which Freud blamed the fantasy of trauma, as opposed to actual trauma, for emotional disturbance in his patients.

But even Freud's modification of his original theory would prove unacceptable to psychiatrists a century later in the 1970s and 1980s. Hypothesizing a biological origin for children's behavioral problems freed psychiatrists from having to deal with the thorny issue of childhood trauma. For a doctor to get a clear picture of trauma from a child is difficult, especially when the parents are present. A child may not disclose trauma for any number of reasons, ranging from fear of consequences to normalizing the experience in the child's mind.

Today, however, we are beginning to recognize that Freud was correct in his view that stressful early experiences are at the root of most psychological problems. Modern research shows that severe stress in early childhood is connected to children's learning problems and behavior problems. Extreme stress even produces changes in the wiring of children's brains. And researchers have found that childhood trauma is more prevalent than was previously thought. Neuroscientist and trauma expert Dr. Bruce Perry says that "by conservative estimates" 40 percent of American children will have at least one traumatizing experience by age eighteen. In 2004 alone, Perry says, an estimated three million reports of child abuse or neglect were made to children's protective services and around 872,000 of these cases were confirmed. However, few researchers have made the connection between the symptoms of psychological trauma and the symptoms of ADHD.

It's worth pointing out that trauma is not always the result of abuse or neglect. Outside of the medical community, the word "trauma" connotes something dramatic and exceptional—abuse or a car crash or the death of a parent, for instance. But the psychiatric definition is much broader. A traumatizing experience, from a developmental standpoint, is a situation that violates our basic understanding of the world and our expectations of how people treat each other. This kind of experience evokes feelings of utter helplessness. Even the most sheltered and protected children witness events or have experiences that can traumatize their consciousness. I have seen children experience nightmares after watching a scary television show or movie before going to bed. Images of car crashes, war, and violence on television, or even classic children's movies such as *Bambi* or *The Lion King*, can be frightening to a four-year-old. A parent's injury, illness, the loss of a job, an affair, or the death of a family member can shatter a child's consciousness and trigger an abrupt change in behavior. For an older child, academic pressure at school, breaking up with a girlfriend or boyfriend, being bullied, or even witnessing a friend being bullied can be a source of traumatic stress.

The Regret of the Biological Psychiatrist

For millions of children, what started as a family feud between biological psychiatrists and psychodynamic-oriented psychiatrists would result in nothing short of disaster. Spitzer and his colleagues, along with the increasingly powerful pharmaceutical industry, created a brave new world that our children would inhabit for decades to come. Yet today, there are expressions of regret. Spitzer has acknowledged that there are no known biological causes for any of the diagnoses in the *DSM-III*, apart from organic disorders (disorders with known biological causes). In a 2012 interview with British psychotherapist James Davies, Spitzer said: "There are only a handful of mental disorders in the *DSM* known to have a clear biological cause. These are known as the organic disorders [such as epilepsy, Alzheimer's, and Huntington's disease]. These are few and far between." When Davies asked, "There are no discovered biological causes for many of the remaining mental disorders in the DSM?" Spitzer replied, "Not for *many*, for *any*! No biological markers have been identified."

Keith Conners, an early advocate for the ADHD diagnosis, has also expressed doubts about the rising ADHD epidemic. In an interview in 2013, Conners called the increasing number of ADHD diagnoses a "national disaster of dangerous proportions." He says the epidemic "is a concoction to justify the giving out of medication at unprecedented and unjustifiable levels." Conners admitted that rating scales like his have "reinforced" the tendency to diagnose ADHD after a mere twenty-minute interview.

Even psychiatrist Allen Frances, the lead author of the *DSM-IV*, has admitted that his own manual cast too wide a net for the ADHD diagnosis, allowing too many children to be diagnosed with a disease they did not have. Of the latest edition of the manual, the *DSM-5*, Frances is bluntly critical. In an article he wrote in the *Huffington Post* on April 14, 2013, "Does DSM-5 Have a Captive Audience?" Frances says: "My advice to clinicians, insurance companies, educators, and policy makers is simply to ignore DSM-5. Its suggestions are reckless, unsupported by science, and likely to result in a great deal of loose, inaccurate diagnosis and unnecessary, harmful, and costly treatment. . . . It is not well done. It is not safe. Don't buy it. Don't use it. Don't teach it."

Apologies are all very well, but the truth is that the *DSM-5* is built on the same shaky paradigm as the third and fourth editions of the manual. And implicit in that paradigm is the mistaken and arbitrary dualism between human being and habitat, as well as the false assumption that psychological problems are best healed by pharmaceutical drugs. So Frances's criticisms of the *DSM-5*—though probably well intentioned because, after all, anyone can change his mind—seem like the pot calling the kettle black. If the ADHD diagnosis had been left out of Frances's *DSM-IV*, the world would be a very different place for America's children.

More than half of the doctors who authored the *DSM-IV* had financial connections to the pharmaceutical industry. One often-quoted study by Lisa Cosgrove and her colleagues found that 95 out of 170 *DSM-IV* panel members had one or more financial ties with drug companies. In Chapter 4, we will look closely at how Big Pharma, working together with Big Psychiatry, fueled the ADHD epidemic.

FOUR

Big Pharma and Biological Psychiatry

> We live in a drug culture, both legal and
> otherwise.
>
> • ELIZABETH WURTZEL

On a rainy evening in the early 1990s, I attended a talk by a child psychiatrist in a large lecture hall at the University of California at Berkeley. I will always remember his talk as the "Ritalin is forever" lecture. The professorial-looking speaker was young, bearded, and well spoken. His words struck me so deeply that I have remembered them all these years. He said that a child diagnosed with ADHD would have to take medication not only during his school years but for his entire life. The psychiatrist compared ADHD to diabetes, and psychostimulant drugs to insulin.

I was stunned, especially since he presented no scientific evidence to support this comparison. I went home and told my husband, a materials scientist with Lawrence Berkeley Laboratory at the time, about the lecture. We both thought the same thing: The psychiatrist was creating a new narrative that would sell more pharmaceutical drugs for kids. He was suggesting that a child born without Ritalin in his blood was suffering from a chronic debilitating illness. It didn't make sense to either of us.

The Kiddie Keystone

In the years following that lecture, the real meaning of what had seemed an absurd analogy between diabetes and ADHD became clear. That Berkeley lecture was just the tip of the iceberg. Academic child psychiatrists were lecturing all across the country, praising the long-term use of stimulant drugs for children and minimizing the drugs' side effects. The Kiddie Keystone drug pipeline was advancing at a breakneck pace. I don't know if the psychiatrist I heard in Berkeley was paid by a pharmaceutical company to give his talk. In light of what we know today, it seems likely that he was.

One of the doctors spreading the message of lifelong Ritalin was a Denver psychiatrist named William W. Dodson. In 2002, Dodson gave a PowerPoint presentation to an audience of physicians in Pasadena, California. Like the psychiatrist in that Berkeley lecture hall, Dodson encouraged the doctors in his audience to "educate" their patients that ADHD was a lifelong disorder and that treatment with stimulant drugs should be long term. Eleven years later, on December 15, 2013, *New York Times* reporter Alan Schwarz wrote an exposé about Dodson's work. The *Times* had obtained a copy of Dodson's presentation and found that his assertions were not supported by "science" since many children "grow out" of behaviors that psychiatrists call ADHD.

Nor did Dodson mention in his lecture that stimulants such as Ritalin and Adderall were "drugs of abuse," which are classified among the most addictive drugs in the medical pharmacopeia. The Drug Enforcement Administration (DEA) classifies Ritalin, Concerta, and Adderall as Schedule II drugs, as addictive and subject to abuse as cocaine and morphine. According to the *Times*, Dodson downplayed other risks of the medication as well. He characterized the side effects of Adderall XR (the once-daily extended-release form of the drug) as "generally mild," despite studies showing that it caused insomnia, appetite suppression and weight loss, adverse cardiovascular reactions, along with rare instances of psychotic episodes. Nonetheless, he minimized the concern about abuse, addiction, and side effects of stimulants, calling these worries "incredibly overblown."

Schwarz reported that Dodson received about $2,000 from Shire, the maker of Adderall, for his Pasadena talk. According to ProPublica, an organization that tracks pharmaceutical company payments to doctors, in 2010–2011, Dodson earned $45,000 in speaking fees from drug companies.

The lectures praising the lifelong benefits of stimulants for children were based largely on the research of one man: child psychiatrist and psychopharmacologist Joseph Biederman of Harvard University and Massachusetts General Hospital. In 1996, the *New York Times* reported that Biederman said (prophetically, as it turned out) that "as many as 10 percent of the nation's children could benefit from Ritalin." Later investigations revealed that Biederman received a substantial amount of funding for his research from pharmaceutical companies. In 2008, a Senate investigation led by Charles Grassley of Iowa found that Biederman had not complied with Harvard's rules about conflict of interest, as he and two colleagues neglected to report $1.6 million paid to them by drug companies.

As reported in the *Boston Globe* on July 2, 2011, Biederman issued a public apology to Harvard and, in addition to other punishment, was placed under a two-year monitoring period during which his speaking engagements were closely watched; nonetheless, his research continued to exert a powerful influence on doctors all over the United States. Every time he mentioned a new ADHD drug in a lecture, thousands of child psychiatrists and pediatricians started writing prescriptions for it. Keith Conners called Biederman "unequivocally the most published psychopharmacology maven for ADHD." Biederman's influence is still evident today by the widespread acceptance by the medical community of medicating children with psychotropic drugs. Not surprisingly, child psychiatry's bent to diagnose and medicate kids for ADHD has sparked a striking increase in the incidence of ADHD diagnoses.

The Marriage of Big Pharma and Big Psychiatry

How did ADHD and stimulant drugs come to gain such an unprecedented hold on us? How did we come to believe, as the prominent psychiatrist Edward Hallowell once claimed, that amphetamines are "safer than aspirin" for our kids? To answer these questions, we need to explore two critical issues: a) how the unholy alliance between Big Pharma and influential academic child psychiatrists came to be so powerful, and b) how Big Pharma and Big Psychiatry managed to seduce the hearts and minds of the American public so that ADHD and stimulant drugs have become part of our national character. We need to understand what made the host population in America so vulnerable to the virus that pharmaceutical companies and academic psychiatrists were spreading.

The psychiatrist who spoke that evening in Berkeley was expressing the new perspective of the *DSM-III*, which claimed ADHD was a biological condition requiring lifelong treatment with medication. As I mentioned earlier, psychiatry had always recognized that children's hyperactive behavior could result from physical causes—including brain injury, diseases such as encephalitis, structural neurological defects, and various poisons. The resulting conditions were called "mild" or "minimal" brain damage. To reduce stigma, this label was later changed to "minimal brain dysfunction," or MBD. But ADHD, and its recommended lifelong treatment with stimulant drugs, was an entirely new way of thinking about hyperactivity and inattentiveness in children who did not have a history of brain damage. To understand how the medical community came to believe that stimulant medications actually corrected biological brain dysfunctions, we must go back more than half a century to 1931 and the work of a pediatrician named Charles Bradley.

A Devoted Pediatrician

Charles Bradley came from a prominent New England family. Following graduation from Harvard Medical School and a residency in neurology at Babies Hospital in New York, he became the director of the Bradley Hospital in Providence, Rhode Island. Founded in 1931 by Charles's great-uncle George Bradley, it was the first hospital in the country devoted to children with neurological and behavior disorders. Originally called the Emma Pendleton Bradley Home, the hospital was named after George Bradley's only child, Emma. Emma was stricken at age seven with encephalitis, which caused massive swelling in her brain. She survived but was left mentally retarded and suffering from cerebral palsy and epilepsy.

Emma's parents wanted to help children with similar conditions and purchased thirty-five acres of peaceful woodland in East Providence, overlooking Narragansett Bay. They built a stately facility in which colonial-style brick buildings dotted the campus, surrounded by open fields for children's sports, scouting activities, and outdoor play in a natural setting. The hospital provided schooling for the children by specially trained teachers who worked with their pupils individually and in small groups. According to the terms of George Bradley's will— the Bradley home opened some twenty years after his death—the facility gave preference to poor children. Families were to be billed only if they had the means to pay.

When Charles Bradley arrived at the Bradley Hospital in 1933, he found children with a wide variety of behavioral and neurological problems, ranging from educational disabilities to neurological conditions, including epilepsy. There were also children with intellectual deficiencies and specific reading disabilities. Some of the children were aggressive and assaultive; others were shy and withdrawn. Bradley set about doing everything he could to minister to the children in his care.

Meanwhile, that same year, far from the gently sloping fields of the Bradley Hospital, a Philadelphia pharmaceutical company called Smith, Kline & French was about to launch a new drug it called Benzedrine. Packaged as an inhaler, Benzedrine was a nervous-system stimulant useful for decongestion of nasal passages. Noticing that the drug had a euphoric effect on patients when they used the inhaler, Smith, Kline &

French began marketing Benzedrine to doctors for use with patients who suffered from mild depression, with favorable results. Soon after, they discovered that Benzedrine also worked as a performance enhancer that improved mental alertness and concentration. Smith, Kline & French was the first company to manufacture an amphetamine drug, and with it came a golden opportunity to develop a wider and more profitable market for Benzedrine.

The ability of Benzedrine to improve mental alertness would make it especially useful to the military in World War II. The Germans used an amphetamine called Pervitin (similar in chemical composition to present-day Adderall) to keep their pilots alert during their blitzkriegs in 1939. Some people even attributed the success of the blitzkriegs to the drug. The British and United States militaries soon began their own experiments with amphetamines and found that the drugs helped pilots stay awake and concentrate, especially on long missions. They began including packages of Benzedrine pills ("bennies") in the kits of every bomber pilot.

In the 1930s, Smith, Kline & French began providing a free supply of Benzedrine to interested doctors, hoping to find new markets. That's how Benzedrine reached Charles Bradley. He hoped the drug would relieve the severe headaches children suffered after a medical procedure to discover brain lesions. He believed the headaches were caused by the loss of spinal fluid during the procedure and hoped that since Benzedrine was a nervous system stimulant, it might stimulate the brain to produce spinal fluid. He found that the drug didn't do much for the children's headaches, but, unexpectedly, it had a dramatic impact on their school performance and their behaviors.

"Arithmetic Pills"

Bradley decided to take a closer look at the effects of Benzedrine on his young charges. In the first of his studies, of the thirty children (twenty-one boys and nine girls) who were medicated with Benzedrine, one half (fifteen students) showed increased motivation to do their schoolwork. As Bradley put it, "there appeared to be a definite 'drive' to accomplish as much as possible during the school period." Speed of reading comprehension and accuracy were also increased, and Bradley noticed changes in social behavior as well. Half the children who had been noisy, irritable, and aggressive became more placid and easygoing. Their mood swings diminished. Some children noticed their own improvement and called Benzedrine "arithmetic pills."

Bradley believed that when a child did not have a biological brain condition, the child's misbehavior, unhappiness, or hyperactivity was due to emotional stress. He therefore designed the hospital as a natural, healthy, and encouraging social environment, in contrast, he believed, to the children's families where the children often relapsed after being released from the hospital.

In 1940, Bradley and his colleague Margaret Bowen published an article in the *American Journal of Orthopsychiatry*, describing a controlled study of amphetamine therapy they had performed with one hundred children at the Bradley Hospital. Their conclusion was intriguing. Although amphetamines could calm the behavior of hyperactive children and improve their school performance while they were taking the drug, the authors argued that drug therapy should not be the preferred treatment for hyperactive and behavior disordered children. Since they believed environmental stressors were the root of these children's problems, the diagnostic process involved identifying these stressors. Residential treatment at the school was a step toward "removing the sources of conflict."

Nor, Bradley argued, could drugs replace psychotherapy as a pathway to permanent mental health. In his view, psychotherapy helped a child to "work out his emotional problems" and trained him to deal with future difficulties. Drugs, on the other hand, do not give the child "the insight into his difficulties which enables him to handle them competently," nor do the drugs train him to deal with future difficulties on his own. In Bradley's opinion, amphetamine therapy for children should be a last resort—only if a child's distressing environment cannot be altered and when effective psychotherapy is not available. And, if the drug must be used, Bradley emphasized that it should be administered only under the supervision of a doctor trained in pediatrics and child psychotherapy.

Bradley also found that the amphetamines sometimes produced "unpleasant and disconcerting" side effects in the children, including insomnia, appetite loss, nausea, dizziness, and fearfulness. One boy became terrified of death after taking the amphetamine, although he had not shown symptoms of fearfulness before. A considerable portion of the children in the studies began experiencing fine tremors of the extremities, especially the hands, which persisted during the entire period of treatment.

Bradley's findings reinforced Smith, Kline & French's conclusion that Benzedrine was a performance enhancer that could raise children's academic achievement. But Bradley had made another observation: The improvement appeared on the first day the amphetamine was given and disappeared on the first day it was discontinued, indicating that the drug did not fundamentally change behavior and performance but only temporarily modified it. Thus amphetamines, though they might help a child focus on an arithmetic test, did not cure the underlying cause of the child's behavioral problems. Later studies have shown that long-term use of amphetamines does not continue to boost academic performance or behavior over and above the child's initial improvement.

Though Bradley's training had been in pediatrics, his work with children at the hospital inspired him to pursue his interest in child psychotherapy. In 1948, he left Rhode Island, where he had lived all of his life, to found the department of child psychiatry at the University of Oregon Medical School, known today as Oregon Health and Science University.

What of Bradley's influence on Smith, Kline & French? According to Yale medical historian Madeleine Strohl, in an article published in the *Yale Journal of Biology and Medicine*, "SKF officials ignored Bradley's work because it focused on children with brain defects, and the company wanted to market the drug to a larger audience of healthy schoolchildren." Strohl argues, too, that in the 1930s, the public criticized giving amphetamines to students for performance enhancement. But Bradley's work did open the door for biologically oriented psychiatrists to associate children's behavioral symptoms of hyperactivity with biological brain problems, since the symptoms of both kinds of problems had responded to amphetamines in Bradley's experiments. Ironically, Bradley's research had the exact opposite effect of what he had hoped.

Defining the Disorder by the Drug

Child psychiatrist Maurice Laufer succeeded Bradley as director of the Emma Pendleton Bradley Home. In 1957, in what turned out to be a pivotal moment in the history of drug treatment of children, Laufer and his colleague Eric Denhoff published an article in the *Journal of Pediatrics* in which they claimed that a favorable response to amphetamines supported a diagnosis of "hyperkinetic disorder of childhood" or "hyperkinetic impulse disorders," terms Laufer coined. Laufer described the hyperkinetic pattern of behavior as characterized by short attention span, poor powers of concentration, and impulsiveness.

Doctors had long recognized that this pattern of behavior could result from physical causes such as encephalitis, which became an epidemic during World War I and left a number of children with true brain damage called "postencephalitic disease." In 1902, the British physician George Still described hyperactive and impulsive behaviors in children that resulted from brain tumors, meningitis, epilepsy, or head injury. Laufer pointed out that these same symptoms could result from emotional causes. Even a nervous system disturbance in the child, he speculated, might be brought about by purely emotional and social factors. Amphetamines helped in most cases, whether the underlying cause of the hyperkinetic behavior pattern was biological or emotional.

Laufer and Denhoff recommended treating hyperkinetic children with amphetamines to calm their behavior and boost their academic work even if they did not have organic brain damage—at least until the children "outgrew" this mode of behavior over the course of time, as was the case with some of the children under their observation.

This was the beginning of the critical paradigm shift in American child psychiatry that I discussed earlier. A diagnosis with a known biological cause, brain damage from disease (postencephalitic syndrome, meningitis, brain tumor), was now merged with the diagnosis of hyperkinetic reaction of childhood merely because the symptoms of both conditions responded to the same drug treatment. Hyperkinetic impulse disorder became defined solely by a drug that decreased behavioral symptoms. The identification of disorders depending on the effective drug treatment was to become a key component of the shift from the psychoanalytic paradigm to biological psychiatry. The Wash. U. trio and other early proponents of biological psychiatry were greatly influenced, directly or indirectly, by the work of Laufer and Denhoff.

One of the curious myths psychiatrists have perpetuated is that if a child does not have ADHD, stimulant medication will not improve his concentration. I've heard this from many parents, who heard it from their doctors. But this claim does not hold up to scientific scrutiny. A 1978 study published in the respected journal *Science* found that stimulant drugs improved attention and focus in "normal" boys as well as in boys who had been diagnosed with ADHD. This study was conducted by Judith Rapoport, a researcher at NIMH. The study challenges the view that if a child has a positive response to stimulants, the child must have ADHD. Indeed, college students and pilots have known for more than half a century that stimulant drugs enhance their alertness and focus. Studies estimate that today as many as 35 percent of college students take prescription stimulants illicitly, without having an ADHD diagnosis.

Where Laufer and Denhoff had opened the door a crack to biological explanations and pharmaceutical treatment, by 1980 that crack had widened to a crevasse. To the biologically oriented research psychiatrists, medication of children for hypothesized biological causes now took on a central role in creating diagnoses that would respond to drug treatment.

To biological psychiatrists, searching for underlying causes for hyperactivity and attention problems in a child's social environment seemed messy and unscientific. Psychiatrists were not comfortable with asking questions about a child's home life. Gone was the golden grain of Bradley's painstaking work—his conviction that medication should be only an adjunct and a last resort for treating troubled children. What the biological psychiatrists saved from Bradley's efforts was merely the chaff—that amphetamines could control kids' behavior and boost their school performance.

Biological psychiatry encouraged clinicians to attribute all behavioral symptoms of children to faulty biology, thus preparing the way for drug companies to take center stage in child psychiatry. And of course, drug companies were ready. The dream of medicating large numbers of healthy children with amphetamines was about to come true.

Protests

This radical change in the hyperactivity paradigm was met with protest from many quarters. One criticism appeared in an especially moving article published in 1978 in *American Educator*, the journal of the American Federation of Teachers, by British sociologist Steven Box. In the article, which was titled "Hyperactivity: The Scandalous Silence," Box charged that using "medical solutions" for kids' behavior problems was a cover for the real reasons these children suffered. "Instead of recognizing the inarticulate cries of rage and despair and examining the very serious problems these hyperactive children face, there is an intense drive to individualize their problems and blame them on organic impairments," he wrote. "Drugs are then administered to dampen and confuse the child's scarcely heard protests."

Box's cogent observation echoed the ideas of the French philosopher and mental health historian Michel Foucault, who contended that framing an emotional problem as a medical condition "silences the patient's story" and distances the doctor from the patient's experience. From my own work with children in therapy, I agree with Foucault. This silencing and distancing were tragic effects of psychiatry's paradigm shift from understanding personal narratives to running through checklists of symptoms. Stuart Kirk and Herb Kutchins, authors of *Making Us Crazy*, mounted their own protests from within the academic mental health community, launching a storm of opinion pieces in newspapers before their book was published in 1997.

The Ghost in the Journal

The new biological psychiatry ignored its critics and continued to be romanced by the whirlwind courtship of drug companies. Pharma showered psychiatrists with grants and substantial funding of buildings for their research (for example, the Johnson and Johnson Center for the Study of Pediatric Psychopathology at Massachusetts General Hospital), opportunities for publication in prestigious journals (the articles were often ghostwritten by advertising agencies hired by drug companies), and lavish vacations and restaurant meals.

The practice of drug companies ghostwriting articles in medical journals dates as far back as the 1950s. In 1959, Tennessee senator Estes

Kefauver launched an investigation by the Senate Subcommittee on Antitrust and Monopoly into questionable drug company practices. Former acting medical director of a division of Pfizer, Dr. Haskell Weinstein, testified before the subcommittee that drug companies ghostwrote many of the journal articles that described their drugs as effective. According to Weinstein, many so-called medical scientific papers were ghostwritten by medical writers employed by the drug company and sent to a journal that relies on the drug company for advertising revenue, "and rarely is publication refused." The papers were slanted to make the drug companies' products look good, with little mention of side effects. On the topic of the targeting of doctors by drug company marketing, Weinstein testified: "The entire promotion and advertising program has been directed at the physician in recognition of his special role. He has been taught, one might almost say brainwashed, to think of the trademark name of the drug at all times. Even new disease states have been invented to encourage the use of some drugs."

One example of ghostwriting occurred in 2002, when Novartis was trying to market its product Ritalin LA, a once-a-day medicine for ADHD. As the sales of this drug began to slide, Novartis had to show that its own version of Ritalin, which had an eight- or nine-hour impact, was better than the twelve-hour action of a competitor's drug. Novartis took the problem to IntraMed, a medical education company owned by the global advertising company WPP. Novartis had no comparative research data to prove its claim about the superiority of Ritalin LA.

Nonetheless, IntraMed hired two academic psychiatrists to "author" the article and told them it wanted a "quick, down and dirty" write-up of the benefits of Novartis's Ritalin LA. The *New York Times* named these doctors as John S. Markowitz and Kennerly S. Patrick of the Medical University of South Carolina. One of IntraMed's ghostwriters, Linda Logdberg, wrote the article, based on an outline approved by IntraMed. Later she began to have misgivings. As the parent of two active children, Logdberg disagreed with Novartis's claim that a drug that worked for eight or nine hours, whose effects wore off right around dinnertime, was better than a longer-acting form of Ritalin.

Logdberg asked to speak with the doctors who were to "author" the article to ask them their views on the drug's benefits. Her IntraMed contact responded with a curt "Just write it." Logdberg claimed her ghostwriting created a fraudulent product; it was "marketing masquerading as science." From her point of view, this advertising posing as medical authorship threatened the fundamental assumptions of scientific research. IntraMed, however, insisted that they merely made "editorial suggestions" and that "the doctors are the ultimate writers." Logdberg disagreed. She gave up ghostwriting soon after writing the article (it was never published) and agreed to be interviewed by Melody Petersen of the *New York Times*. The *Times* reported that a 1998 survey of named authors writing for some of the nation's top medical journals, including the *Journal of the American Medical Association*, found that 11 percent of the articles had been ghostwritten. Some experts think the practice "continues to grow, even as the best journals take steps to prevent it." Whether the editorial boards of most medical journals knowingly make the decision to publish ghostwritten articles is difficult to determine.

Besides hiring advertising companies to secure ghostwriters for journal articles, pharmaceutical companies sponsored conferences at luxurious hotels and resorts, where they "educated" doctors about their products. Forest Laboratories, the maker of the antidepressant Lexapro, hires IntraMed and other advertising companies to organize expensive dinners where research on Forest products is discussed.

The AMA Abandons Its Watchdog Role

Drug companies also buy expensive advertising space in medical association journals. Although drug companies had always advertised in journals, their financial commitment began to escalate in the 1950s. Previously, the American Medical Association had a Seal of Acceptance program for advertisements that appeared in their prestigious journal. The claims of advertisements had to be approved by a committee of distinguished doctors. However, pharmaceutical companies were critical of the restraints imposed on them by the program. As a result of Pharma's discontent and the AMA's budget problems, the program was dropped in 1955. In 1950, drug companies paid the American Medical Association $2.6 million for journal advertisements. By 1960, the amount had climbed to $10 million, which included advertisements and the sale of the AMA's mailing lists. In 2003, drug companies spent $448 million on advertising in medical journals overall. Most drug companies, such as Eli Lilly, AstraZeneca, GlaxoSmithKline, and Merck & Co., marketed directly to doctors by having their sales reps make personal visits to doctors' offices.

Having successfully won over child psychiatrists, Pharma then turned its attention to pediatricians. Since 1979, Pharma has been placing full-page advertisements for stimulants in *Pediatrics*, the official journal of the American Academy of Pediatrics. Pharma also supplied substantial funding to the academy. They hired pediatricians as consultants and speakers, gave them research grants, and awarded them with honoraria. In 2011, the American Academy of Pediatrics issued new guidelines for the ADHD diagnosis, extending it to the preschool crowd. The academy recommended that children as young as four—down from age six—could be diagnosed and medicated for ADHD, without any substantiated biological cause being present.

Although the FDA has not approved methylphenidates for use in children under the age of six, the academy's new guidelines endorsed "off label" prescribing of the drugs to treat younger children. "Off label" use is prescribing a drug for a purpose not approved by the Food and Drug Administration. Pediatrician Mark Wolraich was the chairman of the American Association of Pediatrics subcommittee on ADHD that recommended the new guidelines. According to *New York Times* reporter Roni Caryn Rabin, Dr. Wolraich was a paid consultant to four drug companies that sell ADHD drugs, including Eli Lilly and Shire. According to Rabin, "He said he was compensated for providing expert advice on how the medications could be improved for children's use." Dr. Wolraich recommended that behavioral interventions should be tried first for younger children. If these interventions did not work, however, pediatricians should consider "off label" use of methylphenidates.

Strawberry Speed

Drug giant Pfizer was conveniently positioned to seize on the academy's decision to lower the age limit for the ADHD diagnosis. Pfizer had already been conducting clinical trials of a new oral suspension form of ADHD medication for children too young to swallow pills. This was the fruit-flavored liquid methylphenidate Quillivant XR, approved by the FDA in 2012. Quillivant XR, as a reminder, is a Schedule II federally controlled substance that bears a warning that it can be abused or lead to dependence and may cause psychotic symptoms.

Fortunately for our country's children, not all pediatricians follow the trend of medicating children. One East Coast pediatrician was moved to write to me after he read one of my articles. He thanked me for speaking out about the issue and said he "deplored" the use of psychoactive drugs in children and felt everything should be done to prevent this practice in the United States. Other pediatricians have written to me to express similar feelings of outrage about diagnosing and medicating children for normal childhood behaviors or responses to real problems in their lives.

We Can Make Your Child "More Normal"

Having won over child psychiatry and the American Academy of Pediatrics, Pharma then turned its attention to parents. Drug companies voluntarily respected a United Nations convention and were not yet advertising controlled substances directly to consumers. However, drug companies managed to get parents' attention by distributing pamphlets to schools, a tactic that allowed them to go through professional educators instead of marketing directly to parents. School psychologists, teachers, and school principals, in turn, sent the pamphlets home to parents whose kids were struggling in the classroom. The pamphlets assured parents that the medicine (Ritalin) would not "drug" or "alter the brain" of the child. Rather, Ritalin would make the child more "normal" and allow him to behave better at school. Of course, the fact that the medicine was a Schedule II controlled substance, in the same category as cocaine and OxyContin, was never mentioned.

In 2012, I met one of these parents, Susan Parry, who asked me to speak at the annual conference of the International Society for Ethical Psychology and Psychiatry, an organization that opposes pharmaceutical therapy except for short-term use for severely disturbed adults. Susan said teachers and school counselors had been telling her for years that her feisty son was an "underachiever" and not working up to his potential. Finally, the school recommended testing for ADHD. Susan and her husband, Michael, took their son to various experts for testing, but the results were conflicting and inconclusive.

Watching their son struggle under the pressure of his school's high academic expectations, Susan and Michael eventually decided to put him on Ritalin. Their decision was based on what they read in a pamphlet given to them by a caring teacher who seemed to have genuine concern for their son. The fifteen-page pamphlet was called "Attention Deficit-Hyperactivity Disorder and Learning Disabilities: Booklet for the Classroom Teacher." The author of the pamphlet was Larry Silver, MD, a clinical professor of psychiatry at Georgetown University Medical Center in Washington, DC. The Parrys believed that Dr. Silver was the sole author of the pamphlet—they had no reason to think otherwise. Only later did they notice the small logo on the back. Novartis (formerly called Ciba-Geigy) is the manufacturer of Ritalin and other ADHD drugs.

The Ritalin did help their son's academic performance, but three years later, when he experienced sleep problems and heart palpitations, the Parrys quickly took him off the drug. They were pleased to see that his school performance did not suffer. Perhaps he had simply gained the maturity necessary to keep up with his classmates, or perhaps his teachers' perceptions of him as an "underachiever" had changed. Now Susan and Michael believe that their son never had

ADHD at all. They feel like they were talked into the diagnosis by their son's school with the help of Novartis's propaganda.

Susan has become active in educating parents about the risks of Ritalin and other stimulant drugs. She speaks at conferences and parent groups about her experience and is on the board of the international organization that invited me to its meeting. A *New York Times* article quotes Susan saying that she and her husband felt "seduced, enticed," and "baited" by Novartis.

CHADD

But there are many parents who embrace the ADHD diagnosis for their children. These parents have found that ADHD medications make a world of difference in their children's academic performance and social behavior. By the late 1980s, parents began to flock to advocacy groups, especially to an organization called CHADD—Children and Adults with Attention-Deficit/Hyperactivity Disorder—which was cofounded in 1987 by child psychologist Harvey Parker. A year later, in 1988, CHADD received a donation from drug giant Ciba-Geigy. According to a 1995 PBS *Merrow Report,* "Attention Deficit Disorder: A Dubious Diagnosis?," CHADD established a history of distributing misleading information to hundreds of thousands of parents and teachers to exaggerate the benefits and minimize the side effects of drug therapy, including treatment with Ritalin. CHADD advertised that ADHD was a "chemical imbalance," which Ritalin could correct by increasing the chemical dopamine. The increase of dopamine would make the child's brain more "normal." As I will show in Chapter 5, many experts have challenged this hypothesis.

Early on, Ciba-Geigy was discreet about its role in CHADD, and most parents who joined CHADD did not know about the company's involvement. At a talk I gave in a public library in 1995, a few parents in the audience vehemently protested when I mentioned that Ciba-Geigy had provided money for CHADD. They insisted it simply wasn't true. I think these parents truly believed CHADD was a grassroots parent organization that had their best interests, not those of drug companies, at heart.

Drug giant Shire also saw in CHADD an opportunity to extend the market for its pet ADHD drug, Adderall, and quickly jumped into the funding game. Shire paid CHADD $3 million from 2006 to 2009. Whether intentionally or not, CHADD became a powerful proponent for stimulant drugs. It handed out pamphlets supplied by drug companies to newcomers at meetings, and presented its movie, *ADD and Loving It*, on college campuses all over the country. It produced videos to show to parents. The pamphlets, videos, and movie proclaimed the beneficial effects of stimulants. CHADD provided such a conduit for Ritalin that in 1995, the United Nations International Narcotics Control Board charged CHADD with being a vehicle for marketing a controlled substance directly to the public. In the *Report of the International Narcotics Control Board for 1995*, the board stated, "Treatment of ADD with Ritalin is being actively promoted by an influential 'parent association' that has received significant financial contributions from the leading manufacturer of this preparation in the United States."

The International Narcotics Control Board requested that the authorities of the United States carefully monitor future developments in the diagnosis of ADD in children and the extent to which methylphenidate and other stimulants are used to treat ADD, "in order to ensure that these substances are prescribed in accordance with sound medical practice." The DEA acknowledged that CHADD's financial ties to Ciba-Geigy "may be contrary to international treaty obligations." However, the DEA didn't do much except issue a warning to CHADD that it would use the information it had learned at a later date. CHADD responded by denying that it promoted the use of Ritalin.

In 1996, wanting to avoid adverse publicity, CHADD withdrew its petition to the DEA to reclassify Ritalin from a Schedule II to a Schedule III controlled substance. CHADD had argued in its petition that reports of Ritalin abuse were not evident and that the drug causes only low or moderate levels of dependence. The DEA carefully controls production quotas of Schedule II drugs because these drugs have a high potential for abuse and are likely to be used illegally. Reclassifying Ritalin to a Schedule III substance would have allowed drug companies to increase production of the drug since it would not be subject to the strict quotas. Reclassifying would also have allowed prescriptions for Ritalin to be filled without mandatory visits to the doctor's office, thus making the drug more available.

Not content with advertising their products through schools and CHADD, pharmaceutical companies turned their attention to consumers. At present, there are only two countries in the world that allow direct-to-consumer advertising of prescription drugs: the United States and New Zealand. Other countries have strict laws prohibiting this practice, despite the efforts of Pharma and lobby groups to overturn these prohibitions in Canada and countries in the European Union. However, American pharmaceutical companies refrained from advertising drugs that were controlled substances directly to consumers because of a treaty against this practice signed by the United States. In 1971, the United Nations adopted the Convention on Psychotropic

Substances, which prohibited public advertising of controlled substances. The United States signed the convention, but unfortunately it did not pass any laws supporting the prohibition. For three decades, the pharmaceutical industry voluntarily respected the spirit of the convention. They did not advertise drugs that were stimulants or other controlled substances directly to the public.

Give Me the Grape!

In 2001, the American drug industry changed its mind. In search of even greater profits, it decided to bypass the convention. Drug companies began advertising stimulant drug treatments for adults and children directly to consumers by placing ads for their products in magazines. When these companies were called on the carpet by the DEA, lawyers for the drug companies vowed to defend themselves under the First Amendment right to freedom of speech. The Department of Justice was unwilling to test the case in court. With no law to stop them, drug companies placed expensive full-page color advertisements in popular magazines, especially women's and parenting magazines such as *Family Circle*, *Woman's Day*, and *Redbook*, and *ADDitude* magazine (a publication of CHADD) contained an ad touting a flavored, chewable form of methylphenidate with the slogan, "Give me the grape." Pharma promised magazines even more advertising revenue if they published articles that portrayed the companies' drugs in a positive light. The United States became the only nation to violate the UN convention, and now it consumes a large percentage of the world's stimulant drugs.

Sunshine Act Clouds Pharma's Hopes

In recent years, the marriage of Big Pharma and doctors has been growing stale. There are even signs of imminent divorce. The Physician Payment Sunshine Act, initiated by Senator Charles Grassley, became law in 2013. The Sunshine Act requires pharmaceutical and medical device companies to track and report information on all their interactions with physicians, including payments that relate to medical research.

In the face of pressures from the Sunshine Act and congressional scrutiny of Pharma's practices—including numerous fines for fraudulent advertising—drug companies are rethinking some of their policies. In December 2013, GlaxoSmithKline announced that it will no longer pay doctors to promote its products (*New York Times*, December 16, 2013). Glaxo also agreed to stop tying its sales representatives' compensation to the number of prescriptions doctors write for their drugs. Glaxo's CEO, Andrew Witty, said the changes were part of the company's effort "to try and make sure we stay in step with how the world is changing." The announcement came at a sensitive time for Glaxo. According to the *Times*, the drug giant was under investigation for bribery in China, "where authorities contend the company funneled illegal payments to doctors and government officials in an effort to lift drug sales."

More Regrets

Along with drug companies, many prominent psychiatrists who initially encouraged the rampant diagnosing of ADHD and the use of pharmaceutical therapy are now backpedaling. Psychiatrist Edward Hallowell is the author of the 2011 best seller *Driven to Distraction* and several other highly successful books on the topic of ADD and ADHD. These include *Delivered from Distraction* (1994), *Superparenting for ADD* (2008), and *Answers to Distraction* (2010). Hallowell's books strongly promoted the ADHD diagnosis and treatment with stimulants for both children and adults. But today he says he regrets telling parents that stimulants were "safer than aspirin" and promises he will stop saying so. A 2013 *New York Times* article quotes Hallowell expressing regret for his cavalier recommendations of stimulants: "I hate to think I have had a hand in creating that problem." He also acknowledges that ADHD diagnoses are being made in "slipshod" fashion, and he pointed out the dangerous trend of kids using stimulants as "mental steroids."

A Changing Landscape for Children

Given the arguments I've outlined so far, should any children be medicated for ADHD? I believe that for children who have undisputed brain damage from disease or head injury, prescribing stimulant medications to help them learn in school may be a reasonable decision since there may be no other known way to address the condition. For children without actual brain damage from classical causes such as encephalitis, meningitis, cerebral palsy, brain tumor, epilepsy, or head injury, I propose that instead of relying on a checklist of *symptoms*, doctors, in consultation with social workers or child therapists, use a checklist of possible *causes* of the child's symptoms. These are:

1 • Adverse childhood experiences such as physical or sexual abuse, or neglect. The doctor must determine whether the child's family has a history with children's protective services.

2 • Inappropriate discipline or absence of discipline

3 • Chaotic and disorganized home

4 • A parent's illness, injury, loss of employment, or chronic unhappiness

5 • Unhealthy diet

6 • Excessive screen time

7 • Divorce or chronic marital problems

8 • Conflict with a teacher or boredom in the classroom

9 • Insufficient sleep on an ongoing basis

10 • Insufficient physical exercise

11 • Misinterpretation of a child's normal behavior during a developmental phase

If a child is having problems after the cause or causes have been addressed through interviews with the pediatrician or child psychiatrist,
then family therapy, individual therapy, and/or parent-training classes
should be prescribed. If none of these solves the problems, the doctor
should consult with colleagues before prescribing psychiatric medication and only for children older than six. I am confident that if the
actions I propose become standard practice, only a tiny fraction of children would be medicated for behavioral and learning problems and
the ADHD epidemic would disappear.

I Can't Behave Because I Have ADHD!

Teachers, too, have experienced increased stress in a world that has
become increasingly frenetic. With overcrowded classrooms, they are

less able to devote time to each child and effectively deal with behavioral problems when they arise. A serious problem for teachers is that an ADHD diagnosis exempts a child from having to take accountability for his behavior. After reading one of my articles, a kindergarten teacher wrote to me: "If one more child looks at me after I discipline or redirect them and says 'But I have ADHD,' I'm going to lose it!" The teacher went on to tell me that her standard response to such children is, "It is not an excuse to misbehave, and you do know right from wrong."

The diagnosis of ADHD, as it is used in America today, is a double-edged sword, for teachers, for parents, and for society. On the one hand, stimulant medications such as Ritalin or Adderall calm children down and make them easier to manage at home and at school. The drugs are cognitive enhancers or, as Hallowell phrased it, "mental steroids." They help kids focus on their schoolwork and boost their grades in the short term. On the other hand, as the kindergarten teacher above lamented, children who have been diagnosed with ADHD blame their misbehavior on the disorder and therefore don't learn how to take control of their actions if they're having a particularly bad day or when their medication starts to wear off in the late afternoon.

During the 1980s and 1990s, the hypothesized biological cause of children's behavior problems was especially welcomed by parents because many of them had experienced the beneficial effects of the new antidepressants. If Prozac could work wonders for mothers or fathers suffering from depression, surely Adderall and Ritalin could work similar miracles for their hyperactive children. Magazine articles, often subsidized by drug companies, were filled with personal stories about children transformed thanks to the power of stimulant medications. With this flood of indirect marketing, along with direct marketing to consumers, beleaguered parents could hardly resist bringing their children into the folds of this grand social experiment.

The diagnosis of ADHD brings the child and his family many privileges and special services. Children diagnosed with ADHD are entitled to extra time on tests, including college entrance exams such as the SAT, and sometimes special classes. In 1991, after extensive lobbying by CHADD, Congress included ADHD as a disability that fell under the Individuals with Disabilities Education Act. A diagnosis of severe ADHD, without any other behavioral disorder being present, could then entitle the child's family to disability benefits. Today, mental illness, including ADHD, has become the leading category of disability in children. Finally, having a medical condition removes the stigma attached to a child. Instead of being labeled naughty, disobedient, disturbed, badly behaved, deviant, or even wicked, the child is seen as suffering from an illness outside of his control.

Mental Health and Culture

As a society, we have grown so comfortable with psychiatric diagnoses such as ADHD that we are apt to forget that mental health categories are tied closely to culture. Every culture defines what is considered normal behavior and anyone who behaves differently is considered deviant or abnormal. Consider how more than sixty years ago, a woman who wore a bikini would be considered morally lax, while today they are the height of fashion. Even though psychiatry is supposed to be based on scientific observation, it is hardly black and white, and mental health categories, unlike categories of somatic illnesses, are far from the objective classifications they purport to be.

A striking example of how cultural beliefs and social forces figured in the invention of new categories of "mental illness" occurred in the nineteenth century, when a prominent Southern physician named Samuel Cartwright described two types of "insanity" peculiar to slaves. He called these new mental illnesses drapetomania and dysaesthesia aethiopica. The first was to be diagnosed whenever a slave attempted to run away. The second was thought to be present when a slave displayed idleness or disrespect for his master's property. Cartwright recommended light whippings as a cure for both ailments.

Today, Cartwright's theories are considered pernicious pseudoscience based on bigotry, but they reveal how social prejudices can become legitimized as "scientific knowledge" and as "real" mental illnesses. Mental health categories are fashioned by particular people and subgroups of society (and the fashioning is not always separate from subjective motives or social fads) at a particular time in history and at a particular place.

But the power and authority of psychiatry, which has grown considerably since Cartwright's time, has lured us into accepting these diagnoses as fact. Although the higher-minded among the creators of psychiatric categories strive to be scientific, the categories they invent are not the result of rigorous scientific thought. They are the outcome of a subjective consensus among panels of psychiatrists who create and codify them in diagnostic manuals whose titles have a scientific and authoritative ring. Though psychiatrists may wish the general public to believe otherwise—and perhaps they even believe it themselves—the psychiatric categories in their "diagnostic and statistical manuals of mental disorders" are the lenses through which we observe nature, not nature itself. The goal of the scientific study of mental illness is, as Plato put it, to "carve nature at the joints." Sadly, however, when nonscientific political motives derail rational thinking, the study of mental illness becomes empty nomenclature, having little resemblance to nature at all.

Who knows? ADHD may one day join the rubbish heap of drapeto-mania, dysaesthesia aethiopica, and many other discarded diagnoses that were eventually exposed for what they were: fads in the collective imagination of certain groups who felt their power threatened or who stood to profit.

Mark Twain famously said, "There are lies, damned lies and statistics." In the social sciences statistically based research findings are inherently fraught with controversy. So how do we choose between studies that have contradictory findings? What are we to think of opposing inter-pretations of research in the popular media? What research can we trust and which studies should we doubt? In the next chapter, I will take a deeper look at these issues.

FIVE

The Message in the Media

> If you don't read the newspaper, you're
> uninformed. If you read the newspaper,
> you're misinformed.
>
> • MARK TWAIN

Most of us would agree with Mark Twain about the stories we read in newspapers. We feel a little skeptical, a little doubtful that we are getting the whole truth. Sometimes, though, newspaper stories can be downright confusing. Consider these two articles about drug treatment for kids diagnosed with ADHD. Both stories were published in highly reputable newspapers. The first appeared in the *Washington Post* on September 21, 2007. The article declared: "ADHD Drugs Help Boost Children's Grades." The second story appeared six years later in the *Wall Street Journal* (July 8, 2013). It announced "ADHD Drugs Don't Boost Kids' Grades." What a difference six years make.

What's going on? Did the facts change? Was the *Wall Street Journal* correcting an earlier error? A little research shows us that the stories are based on two different research studies. The later study contradicted the findings of the earlier study. This is not so unusual. Journalists are quick to report on research that seems to promise new hope for a medical condition. The *Washington Post* story was based on a study that appeared in the respected *Journal of Developmental Behavioral Pediatrics* and was written by several distinguished pediatricians. The researchers found that kids with ADHD who took stimulant drugs did better at school than the control group of ADHD kids who did not take medication. The research team followed 370 children with ADHD from the time they were diagnosed with ADHD to age eighteen. The children who were treated with stimulants took them for three years. They were tested at age thirteen, along with the group of ADHD kids who were not given the drugs. The researchers found that the kids who took the drugs did better in a number of ways.

The study concluded that "stimulant treatment of children with AD/HD was associated with higher achievement in reading, fewer absences from school, and a lower risk of having to repeat a grade." The authors claimed that their research supported long-term medical treatment for children with ADHD. The drugs did not merely control the kids' behavioral symptoms in the short term, but they also improved the children's lives over many years. The medicated kids didn't drop out or skip school as much as the children who didn't receive the drugs.

Who Pays for Research Studies?

The lead author of the study, Dr. William Barbaresi of the Mayo Clinic, was quoted by the *Washington Post* as saying that stimulant medication needs to be considered "for every child with ADHD." When we hear words like these, we must ask, "Who paid for this study?" And we are not surprised to learn that some of the funding came from Johnson & Johnson, the maker of the methylphenidate drug Concerta. Methylphenidate was the drug the researchers used in the study. Additional funding came from the Mayo Clinic and two public health agencies.

The *Washington Post* reported mixed reactions in the medical community to Barbaresi's research. Some doctors thought that the study reinforced what they were already telling parents: Medicating hyperactive and inattentive children had long-term as well as short-term benefits. Other doctors thought that studies about ADHD treatments should not be limited to drugs. What about giving kids more physical activity outdoors, removing highly processed foods from their diets, or decreasing their exposure to media? Yet another group of experts questioned the scientific validity of the study. Can we really trust the researchers' conclusion about the long-term benefits of stimulants in children's lives? Was the study trustworthy? Did the conclusions follow from the data?

Not really, answered neuroscientist François Gonon and his team in a 2008 paper published in *Trends in Neuroscience*. Dr. Gonon is a professor at the University of Bordeaux and a researcher at France's Center for Scientific Research. He is one of a new breed of neuroscientists who conduct research on research (a.k.a. meta-research) by looking closely at the methodology and internal consistency of studies that appear in prominent journals. Gonon is particularly interested in ADHD and how the popular press sensationalizes findings even when the research is deficient or weak. He finds that some studies published in premier journals such as *Science* and the *Lancet* omit facts, misrepresent data, and suffer from internal inconsistencies. When they are written up in the popular press, these flawed studies have powerful impacts on doctors, parents, and ultimately children.

Gonon's group found that the Barbaresi study had a number of serious flaws and didn't really prove what it claimed to prove. For one thing, of the 349 medicated children, only 26 showed improved reading scores. And these children had received especially high daily doses of the methylphenidate, sometimes exceeding 40 mg. (A more typical daily dose is 20–30 mg.) Second, said Gonon, the data gathered in the study did not support the conclusion. In particular, the actual data gathered by the researchers indicated that the improvements in reading scores were similar between the medicated children and the non-medicated kids. Both groups improved in reading at a similar rate. Thus, the treated children did not actually have the advantage claimed in the conclusion. Finally, the Gonon team pointed out that the proportion of school dropouts was about the same between the medicated and non-medicated groups (22 percent versus 25.8 percent). The conclusion that the medicated group enjoyed more benefits over the long term did not really match the data.

Given the weakness of the study's results, Gonon decided the research of Barbaresi and his colleagues actually concluded the opposite of what it claimed; namely, said Gonon, it "supports the view that psychostimulant medication does not improve long-term academic outcomes of ADHD children" since the non-medicated group of ADHD kids improved just as much as the medicated kids.

The MTA Study

Gonon points to other research that questions the notion that stimulants benefit ADHD kids over the long term. One of these studies was the source for the 2013 *Wall Street Journal* article. This major study, funded by the National Institute of Mental Health, was called the Multi-modal Treatment Study of Children with ADHD, abbreviated as the MTA. The MTA was the largest placebo-controlled study of stimulant drugs ever conducted and was funded entirely by the United States government; the researchers received no money from pharmaceutical companies.

Using a sample of 579 children who had been diagnosed with ADHD, the MTA looked at the long-term effects of treatment with methylphenidate drugs. During the first year of the study, eight- and nine-year-olds taking the drugs did perform nominally better than their peers who had not been medicated. However, in a three-year follow-up, the effects of the drugs leveled off, with the medicated and non-medicated students performing equally well. A follow-up eight years later showed no differences between the medicated and non-medicated children on several measures of academic achievement. The MTA team concluded that there were no long-term residual benefits of stimulant treatment of ADHD during childhood. One of the follow-ups also reported that methylphenidate treatment had an impact on children's physical growth. The group of children who received medication showed reduced growth in height compared with the group that was not medicated.

So what are we to make of the MTA? We are not surprised that stimulants helped ADHD-diagnosed kids do better in the short term, although psychiatrist Daniel Carlat, author of *Unhinged: The Trouble with Psychiatry*, was even skeptical about this point. The group of kids in the MTA who took stimulants, Carlat pointed out, were getting more than merely drugs. The kids taking the medications had a higher level of care than a typical ADHD kid receives in a visit to the doctor's office.

The monthly doctor's appointments of children in the study lasted a full half-hour. Doctors provided support and practical advice to the children and gave their parents reading material about ADHD. During these visits the doctors also reviewed information about the child's symptoms from both parents and teachers. That is not typical in a ten-minute medication checkup. Finally, doctors used a research-driven protocol to ensure that stimulant doses for the kids were adjusted to optimum effectiveness. Unfortunately, none of these interventions are typical in the usual treatment of ADHD at the doctor's office.

In comparing outcomes from scientific studies it's important to keep in mind that research moves in a chaotic progression, with new hypotheses and conclusions refuting and replacing older ones all the time. However, research findings about ADHD affect the lives of real children and their families, just as refuted findings in other fields affect the lives of real people. Consider the impact of the *Washington Post* article and the Barbaresi study, along with the media chatter that followed. Since 2007, the number of kids receiving the ADHD diagnosis in the United States has risen 16 percent. About two thirds of these children received prescriptions for stimulant medications. Well-intentioned parents and doctors who read the *Washington Post* article were left with the impression that stimulant drugs would help ADHD kids not only in their short-term school performance but even over the long term. They believed that giving their kids the drugs would reduce absenteeism, prevent their kids from dropping out of high school, and even help them get into a better college or get a better job. This impression resulted in more children receiving prescriptions for stimulants because parents and doctors were led to believe that this was the best way to help them.

Of course, before doctors get out their prescription pads, they usually check the sources of newspaper articles that proclaim exciting new developments in medicine. They don't typically believe what they read in newspapers or on the Internet any more than the rest of us do. However, they do believe they can rely on "scientific" studies that appear in respected peer-reviewed medical journals. They count on the integrity of the peer review process, whereby experts evaluate the work before it is published. With their hectic schedules, doctors do not always have the time to scrutinize studies with the critical eye of a Gonon. Also, wanting to provide quick relief for children who are falling behind at school, doctors can scarcely afford to wait and see if new research verifies or refutes the positive results of a study. They don't have time to read critiques of every new scientific study on ADHD. And of course, like all of us, doctors tend to believe in studies that confirm their existing beliefs and practices.

Journalistic Deficit Disorder

We cannot blame journalists for reporting on initial studies that yield striking conclusions in a hot field. Articles about health sell newspapers and are large influencers of public opinion. In 2012, Gonon and his team wrote a paper called "Why Most Biomedical Findings Echoed by Newspapers Turn Out to Be False: The Case of Attention Deficit Disorder." This article caught the eye of the *Economist* magazine. An *Economist* reporter described Gonon's research in a 2012 article with the interesting title "Journalistic Deficit Disorder." Gonon's group found that forty-seven research papers on ADHD were cited in 347 articles in English-language newspapers during the 1990s. Of the top ten papers, seven claimed to verify novel hypotheses. Of these, the conclusions of six were either completely refuted or substantially weakened by subsequent investigations. The seventh has been neither confirmed nor rejected. This is not unusual, reports the *Economist*. Lots of hypotheses don't stand the test of time. But after reporting the initial discoveries, newspapers lost interest. Very few of them reported the weakening or refutation of the earlier positive findings. It's no surprise that the press has a natural bias toward the novel and exciting. A bit of journalistic attention deficit disorder is only to be expected, says the *Economist*. The public, however, remains misinformed because the results of follow-up studies are not widely disseminated.

Science, however, is a different story. We expect strict integrity from scientific researchers. Unfortunately, this is not always the case. Eight of the ten papers Gonon's group studied appeared in prestigious peer-reviewed medical journals such as the *Lancet* and the *New England Journal of Medicine*. But the follow-ups that weakened the studies' hypotheses were hidden in more obscure journals, which busy doctors were less likely to read.

Gonon warns us that it's not only a matter of maintaining our skepticism as we read news and surf the Web. The scientific papers themselves are rife with weaknesses such as misrepresentation of data and omission of significant facts. In some ways, Gonon and his fellow neuroskeptics resemble Socrates, who was known for his stinging questions that unraveled accepted dogma. Indeed, Socrates convinced so many young people to turn a skeptical eye on dogma that he was put to death by the Athenian government for fomenting unrest.

Lies, Damned Lies, and Medical Science

Another prominent present-day Socrates is Stanford University professor John Ioannidis, who takes Gonon's scrutiny of biomedical research one step further. In 2005, he published a widely influential paper called "Why Most Published Research Findings Are False." Ioannidis worried that the gold standard of science—replication—has become tarnished in today's research environment. Replication is the ability of a researcher to reproduce a research finding from a different study. An example is the Southampton Study in Great Britain which replicated American pediatrician Benjamin Feingold's findings on the negative effects of artificial food dyes on children, thus reinforcing the original hypothesis. (I will discuss Feingold's research and the Southampton Study in Chapter 7.) But in the fiercely competitive struggle to get funding for their research, most scientists are more eager to test their own novel hypotheses than to replicate the results of others.

The *Atlantic*, with a nod to Mark Twain's distrust of scientific research as well as newspapers, published an article about Ioannidis's work entitled "Lies, Damned Lies, and Medical Science," by David H. Freedman. Can medical research really be as bad as that? Afraid so, Ioannidis tells us, and he defends his view with formidable arguments.

Ioannidis offers six reasons why research findings can be false, two of which are especially relevant to our discussion of ADHD. He points out that research findings are less likely to be valid when financial interests are greatest, and also when interest in a particular scientific field is especially intense. Both are true for ADHD. ADHD drugs are a nine-billion-dollar-a-year industry, and the debate about whether ADHD exists at all couldn't be more heated. In a hot field of scientific research, conflicting and contradictory reports follow one another in rapid progression. Ioannidis calls these swiftly changing research findings the "Proteus Phenomenon," after the Greek god of the sea, Proteus, who could instantly change his shape from one form to another.

The sea is changeable but it also reflects. All research, says Ioannidis, reflects the mind-set of the researcher. All medical research contains bias because it is impossible to take the human observer out of the picture. Researchers go into a study wanting certain results and then they get them (if they don't, we never hear about the outcome). Although we think of scientific process as objective and fair-minded, subjective interests and agendas always play a part. First, researchers are obsessed with getting funding. This pressures them to manipulate and distort their data—whether consciously or not—so as to arrive at the finding most likely to earn them funding.

Like Gonon, Ioannidis observes that many eye-catching scientific research findings published in prestigious journals are contradicted by later findings. But even if they are refuted by rigorous studies, if merely one less cautious study proves the original findings to be true, through a clever selection of data, it is this single study that doctors will read about in medical journals and the public will hear about on the evening news.

Furthermore, prejudice toward the correctness of a certain view inevitably prevails in a popular scientific field. This prejudice undermines the predictive value of research findings. Prejudiced stakeholders with strong motivation to put forth a particular worldview can also create a barrier that stands in the way of disseminating results that contradict their position. For example, peer reviewers often depend on drug companies to help fund their research or serve as paid consultants for them. This leads to bias about selecting papers that show positive results for pharmaceutical therapy and suppressing papers that show negative results. Suppression of research can have nonfinancial motivations as well. Prestigious scientists may suppress via the peer review process findings that conflict with their own research or worldview, thus perpetuating false dogma instead of the findings of legitimate science.

According to Ioannidis, one especially protean field is molecular genetics. Genetic research is key in the nature-nurture debate about whether ADHD exists as a real medical entity. There are currently three positions in that debate. The first, the nature hypothesis, states that ADHD is a real illness primarily caused by biological factors such as genetic anomalies. The second is that behaviors that we group together as ADHD stem from a combination of biological and social factors, or genes interacting with the environment. The third position is that ADHD is not a true disease entity or medical condition, but that behaviors our society calls ADHD are caused by social factors such as trauma, poverty, a chaotic family life, too much exposure to electronic screens, and other environmental adversities. Those who maintain this last position, and I am among them, believe that ADHD is a social construct that varies in its definition from culture to culture.

Weak Evidence

Over the past three decades, the American public has been led to believe that the nature hypothesis is correct. In reality, however, the evidence for a genetic cause is fragile and controversial. A major study that promotes a genetic factor in ADHD was conducted by Nigel Williams and a team of British, Icelandic, and Norwegian researchers, and was published in the *Lancet* in 2010. The researchers found that rare chromosomal deletions and duplications were associated with ADHD. In other words, children with ADHD were more likely than other children to have a particular genetic anomaly. The study's conclusion, "ADHD is not purely a social construct," was echoed by several prominent newspapers and other news sources.

The Wellcome Trust, which contributed funds for the study along with several public sources, issued a press release declaring that the research provided "the first direct evidence that attention-deficit hyperactivity disorder is a genetic condition." Not surprisingly, several members of the Wellcome Trust had associations with drug companies that make ADHD medications, including Shire, Pfizer, GlaxoSmithKline, and Eli Lilly. Obviously, drug companies welcome the finding that ADHD is a genetically based biological "disease." If doctors believe ADHD has a genetic cause, they are more likely to prescribe pharmaceutical treatment instead of promoting interventions such as parent-training classes and talk therapy.

Gonon turned his attention to the Williams study and found many flaws. First, of the 366 children diagnosed with ADHD, 33 also had mental retardation. By its very definition, a diagnosis of ADHD excludes mental retardation. The prevalence of the genetic anomalies (alleles, or variants, of the DRD4 gene) in children with ADHD alone was relatively small compared to the control group, 12 percent versus 7.5 percent. This result indicates a risk factor, but scarcely a cause, since 78 percent of the kids diagnosed with ADHD did not have the allele.

To make this point clearer, consider a genuine genetic-based illness such as Down syndrome, in which 100 percent of the children diagnosed have a genetic anomaly, namely an extra copy of chromosome 21. This anomaly is the sole determinant to obtain a diagnosis, and there is a test for it. Behavioral symptoms are irrelevant in the diagnosis. The genetic variation observed in the Williams study is not the cause of ADHD. It is at most merely a potential risk factor. As Gonon points out, the Williams study does not provide even a "hint" of a genetic test to confirm an ADHD diagnosis. The anomaly does not occur in all or even most children with ADHD. A diagnosis of ADHD, says Gonon, is based on an assessment of behavioral symptoms, not on a genetic analysis. This is why the recognition of ADHD is more prevalent in some countries than others; it is widely subject to cultural interpretation.

Gonon was not the only scientist to attack the Williams study. Child psychologist Oliver James criticized the researchers for hyping their findings. He pointed out that "only 57 of the 366 children with ADHD in the study had the genetic variant supposed to be a cause of the illness." Therefore, most ADHD in children must be caused by something other than the genetic anomaly. Another criticism of the Williams study was leveled by Professor Lindsey Kent at the University of St. Andrews in the UK. The impression that the study found a genetic cause for ADHD is misleading, he said. They found *genetic variations* that seem to raise the risk of ADHD. This is a crucial difference.

Kent compares this to cigarettes: Smoking raises the risk of coronary disease, but not everyone who smokes has a heart attack and plenty of people who do not smoke will have one. An article criticizing the Williams study appeared in the *Huffington Post* in 2010 with the title: "Is ADHD Genetic? Study Finds Link to Missing DNA." However, despite its serious weaknesses and flaws, the Williams study has been cited 319 times in scientific journals and in myriad news reports, giving it a vast sphere of influence.

Genes and Environment

In the absence of a consensus among scientists regarding a genetic biomarker for ADHD, many researchers who previously supported the genetic causality theory have started to take a more moderate position, conceding that environmental factors do play a significant role in the expression of genes. In an editorial in the *American Journal of Medical Genetics* Samuele Cortese and his coauthors insist that genetic research has always acknowledged the interaction between genes and environment (even if the researchers never said so). "That environmental factors do play a significant role in the etiology of ADHD is unquestionable," say the authors.

Cortese's group also defends itself against another criticism leveled by Gonon's team, namely that genetic research favors psychiatric drug cures for ADHD. The authors insist, "We do not think that research in the neurobiology of ADHD favors the use of pharmacological treatments." This conclusion seems to fly in the face of the undisputed fact that much of the research into biological causes of ADHD has been funded by pharmaceutical companies. These studies frequently conclude, as Barbaresi's team did, that ADHD drugs should be considered for every child with ADHD. It's of interest that both Stephen V. Faraone and Samuele Cortese accepted consulting fees from Eli Lilly, Shire, and other drug companies.

The Dopamine Hypothesis

In a response to Cortese's defensive editorial, Gonon argued that neurobiological observations are in fact misrepresented to the lay public so as to support stimulant drug treatment for ADHD. For example, the view that a lack of dopamine is the cause of ADHD has been widely circulated in newspapers, with drugs that stimulate dopamine release touted as fixes. These articles are, once again, based on misrepresentations of the actual research findings, which showed only a weak connection between a dopamine deficit and ADHD. Gonon also argues that parents and professionals are more likely to accept genetic theories of ADHD because this viewpoint prevents parents from feeling guilty. Even worse, Gonon finds it tragic that the wide dissemination of these views means that mental health policy makers do not look toward prevention. In the case of excessive TV watching, for example, even though it has been identified as a strong risk factor for ADHD, American public policy shies away from legislative intervention.

When considering genetic causes, one must take into account that heritability studies cannot differentiate between the purely genetic and the interaction of genes and environment. It's encouraging that some genetic determinists now concede that ADHD is caused by "a combination of biological and social factors." It is good to know that the nature proponents are coming around to a rational consensus that environmental factors have some causal role in ADHD. This opens the way for research on how non-pharmaceutical treatments such as family therapy and parent-training classes can be as effective as drug treatment.

Neuroscience Fiction

Today, discoveries in neuroscience, especially in the area of brain imaging, are particularly alluring to the media. There is great public interest in the notion that brain scans allow us to "see" ADHD in the brain and thereby guide us toward diagnosis and treatment. The excitement about what brain scans can or cannot tell us about mental health and behavior has brought forth a new generation of neuroskeptics and neurodoubters.

A *New Yorker* blog post called "Neuroscience Fiction" captures the spirit of the new neuroskepticism. The author of the blog, NYU psychologist Gary Marcus, points out that while brain scans show particular regions of the brain lighting up during various types of activities, these scans don't tell us as much as we think they do. Most of the action in the brain is at the neuron level, not in the larger brain regions that we can see with today's scans. Vast arrays of individual neurons interact in complex behaviors, but brain scans cannot show us how these neurons interact. Simple explanations for complex brain functions make splashy headlines, but they rarely show any relation to behavioral "illnesses." As Marcus puts it, "Neuroscience has yet to find its Newton, let alone its Einstein."

Neuroskeptic Dorothy Bishop

Professor Dorothy Bishop of Oxford University has swept onto the scene as an outspoken neuroskeptic. Like Ioannidis and Gonon, Bishop conducts meta-research in neuroscience. She, too, poses uncomfortable questions about whether neuroscience studies hold up to rigorous scrutiny. In a remarkable 2012 lecture to the Association for Child and Adolescent Mental Health, Bishop demonstrated how brain imaging can lure perfectly rational people into a trance of misinformation. She described a study called "The Seductive Allure of Neuroscience Explanations," in which participants were given both a strong and a weak explanation for a psychological phenomenon. The weak explanation, however, was prefaced with the phrase "Brain scans indicate . . ." Most people found the weak explanation much more convincing. The weakness was "hidden" by the verbiage about what brain scans purportedly proved. "Anything neurosciency," said Bishop, "tends to lead to the loss of our critical faculties." To support this charge, Bishop brought forth one more piece of evidence. She told her audience that when a dead salmon was placed in a brain scanner and asked to "rate" pictures of human emotion, different areas of the dead fish's brain were seen to light up on the scans.

Research scientists, too, seem to fall into a trance when it comes to brain scans. At the same presentation, Bishop discussed a paper written by several eminent authors and published in the prestigious journal *Proceedings of the National Academy of Sciences*. The paper was called "Natural Deficits in Children with Dyslexia Ameliorated by Behavioral Remediation: Evidence from Functional MRI." Children's brains were scanned before and after an intervention that claimed to improve language ability. After the intervention, the children's scans showed increased activity in certain regions of the cortex. Bishop pointed out that the study had significant weaknesses, which even careful researchers overlooked, seemingly because of their fascination with the power of brain scans.

Most striking, the study did not have an untreated control group, an essential part of any well-conducted study. Bishop pointed to four more flaws. The team did not take into account various reasons why children might have done better on the test the second time around—maturation (children's abilities develop over time), the practice effect (when people take a test for the second time, their brains respond differently and their scores improve), regression to the mean (if participants are chosen on the basis of low scores, their scores tend to improve), and the placebo effect (the extra attention alone could have helped the children do better on the second test). Russ Poldrack, one of the authors of the paper, read Bishop's analysis of his study's weaknesses and actually agreed with her. He sent out a widespread tweet saying that Bishop was "spot on" in her critique. Bishop found five other studies in top journals that suffered from similar flaws.

What we learn from neuroskeptics like Dorothy Bishop is not to lose our minds when we are shown images of the brain. In the same vein, a team of British scientists analyzed nearly three thousand articles about neuroscience in the popular press between 2000 and 2010. They found that the media distorted and embellished the findings of the studies on which the articles were based. Much of this "neuropop" has an authoritative ring because people tend to revere any news embellished with the flavor of neuroscience or the glamour of brain images. That is why news about neuroscience, even more than other news, should be taken with a grain of skeptical salt.

These warnings are important, but science must go beyond critique and debunking. There is not yet any universally accepted legitimate research that relates brain imagery to either the diagnosis or treatment of ADHD. Back in the 1930s, children with true brain damage treated by Charles Bradley did better at school when they took amphetamine drugs (their "arithmetic pills"). Today's brain scan proponents are extending the organic brain damage model to justify drugging children on the basis of "organic" problems purportedly "seen" in brain scans.

In the final analysis, all research is statistical. A research study, no matter how scrupulous and free from bias, cannot predict results for any particular person. Each individual has a unique story that ultimately reveals the true reasons for troubled behavior. A child's individual story is both a clue to the cause of his troubles and a signpost that guides us to help him.

When it comes to ADHD-type symptoms, we've seen that parent-training programs have benefited both children and parents. And what of teachers? Do different cultural attitudes toward education and the role of teachers make a difference to ADHD diagnoses in children? In the next chapter I look at schools and education, both in America and abroad. Through the prism of other cultures, we can see more clearly what changes would benefit our own schools and our own children.

PART III

Saving
Our
Children

SIX

Why American Schools Have to Change

We used to have a name for sufferers
of ADHD. We called them "boys."

• ANONYMOUS

If Huckleberry Finn could choose where to go to school today, he
would probably pick Finland, and not just because of his name. In
Finland, Huck wouldn't be tempted to cut school because Finnish
teachers allow children to be children and, most important, they allow
boys to be boys. In Finland, Huck wouldn't even have to start school
until he turned seven. When he started, he would spend only four
hours a day, as opposed to the typical six or seven in America, sitting in
a classroom, and even then not consistently. For every forty-five minutes of lessons, Finnish children get a fifteen-minute break for free play.

After school he could either go home to play with his friends or join
two thirds of Finland's children in an after-school sports association.
He'd even have a free healthy lunch at school. Best of all, he would have
no or very little homework, which he'd probably complete before leaving school for the day. So his afternoons would be free for socializing
and lots of physical exercise, as well as undoubtedly getting into a bit
of harmless mischief.

A boy like Huck—whose mother had died and whose father was the town drunk—would get plenty of special attention at school if his grades started to slip. The school's team of special educators, which include a social worker, a psychologist, and a nurse, would set about finding the best learning solution for him. This might mean special tutoring, or simply giving Huck lots of one-on-one encouragement and support. He might get to sit in the principal's office for part of the day and choose books that caught his interest from the stack on the principal's desk.

In the United States today, a high-spirited boy like Huck Finn undoubtedly would be diagnosed with ADHD, if not bipolar disorder, and given a prescription for one or more psychotropic drugs. But in Finland only 0.1 percent of children take ADHD medication, and Finnish doctors and educators understand that when there is little pressure to rush a child's learning, and no anxious parents demanding Ritalin, children are much more likely to grow out of hyperactivity and inattentiveness.

All the school support services available to Huck would be free. Nearly 30 percent of Finland's children receive some kind of special help during their first nine years of school without being labeled as "delinquent" or "lazy" or diagnosed with ADHD. Guidance and psychological services are available in every school. Teachers, too, are committed to every child's success and give extra help to those who need it.

Finland's schools rank among the best in the world in reading, science, and math, according to the results of respected international testing. In recent years, Finnish students' test scores have lagged a bit behind those of East Asian children, who are known for their exhaustive cramming and rote memorization. But Finland's students still score much closer to the top than American students, whose scores have drifted to the middle of the heap since the 1970s, well below such countries as China, Japan, France, and Canada.

Educational Reforms

Finland did not always lead the pack in school performance. According to Finnish educator Pasi Sahlberg, in the 1960s the Finnish school system was badly in need of reform. Education was inequitable, with children "streamed" into different schools according to their perceived levels of ability after four years of primary education. Influential Finns, including members of Parliament, believed that "everyone cannot learn everything." That is, they thought that talented students from educated families were better learners than less privileged students and that they deserved a greater allocation of the country's education resources.

However, in the late 1960s a spirit of reform was in the air. Growing pressure from both teachers and parents began to influence Finland's social policy. A teachers' association representing nearly 90 percent of Finnish primary school teachers called for a more equitable education system that would accommodate the needs of children from all economic and social classes, not only the needs of children from the elite privileged class. Parents demanded an improved and more comprehensive education for their children. The country initiated a program of educational reform that had stunning results. The core idea was that all students, regardless of their family background, socioeconomic status, or ethnicity, would enroll in the same basic nine-year schools. The implementation of this idea was, according to Sahlberg, nothing short of revolutionary. By 2003, Finland's students scored first in reading and science, second in math, and third in problem solving on the global PISA (Program for International Student Assessment) test.

High Standards for Teachers

Finland also raised its standards for teachers, requiring them to have at least master's degrees. In Finland today, being a teacher is regarded as a highly prestigious and even noble profession. Teachers command top salaries, and master's level programs are highly competitive. Only the top 10 percent of the country's university graduates make the cut for a master's program in teaching. The job description of a teacher in Finland differs from that of their American counterparts. In elementary schools, teachers spend four hours a day in the classroom and the rest of the time assessing their students' progress and providing support to those who need it. Teachers also have time to reflect on their day and talk to other teachers about changes they would like to see in the school curriculum. All teachers spend two hours a week on professional development, with full pay.

In his book *Finnish Lessons: What Can the World Learn from Educational Change in Finland?* Sahlberg writes that the country's overall goal was to have an educated public at large, not merely an educated upper class. "The primary aim of education," he said in an interview, "is to serve as an equalizing instrument for society." In Finland today, schools in nonaffluent areas are as good as those in affluent districts. There are no private schools or private universities in Finland. All schools are publicly financed. Finland also goes against the tide of what we in the United States have considered to be essential in educational reform: core subjects, competition, standardization, and test-based accountability.

Unlike the United States, which starts standardized testing of children as early as third grade, Finland does not test children for the first six years of school. Finnish teachers don't have the stress of "teaching to the test" or knowing they will be judged by their pupils' test scores. Finnish early education is about helping each child discover his interests and abilities, and educators there believe all pupils can learn if given the proper opportunities and support. The goal is to design learning environments that enable different kinds of learning for pupils from diverse backgrounds.

Finland's view that teachers must learn to vary their teaching styles to reach diverse students with different strengths and needs resonates with my experience. During graduate school, I taught college classes mainly to middle-class and upper-middle-class students at private colleges. Then one day a friend asked me to fill in for her for a semester at the community college in downtown Chicago where she taught humanities. On the first day of class, I was struck by two things. First, as a Caucasian I was a minority of one. Second, I was going to have to come up with new methods of teaching kids who hadn't been taught to write well in high school. I changed from written assignments and tests to spoken ones. I took the students on field trips to the Art Institute and to high-quality movies. The students gained self-confidence and were more willing to speak up and share their opinions. Teaching them Shakespeare's *Hamlet* was a joy, for I found that these students had an extraordinary grasp of the family dynamics beneath the story. By the end of the semester, class attendance had improved and all of the students earned passing grades. Rising to the challenge of teaching this diverse group of students was so satisfying that I signed up for another semester.

The United States cannot adopt Finland's model directly, since we have a much larger and more diverse population than that small Scandinavian country (its population is similar to that of Maryland or Oregon) where only 5 percent of the total population of 5.5 million is foreign born. But we should at least take some lessons from their example. Our American education system is currently based on inequality, just as Finland's was in the 1960s. In the United States, rich and upper-middle-class kids have access to the best schools, the best teachers, and later, the best private universities. To go against this entrenched elitist value system in the name of having a more educated society would ruffle many feathers. But, as we will see later in this chapter, some respected and innovative thinkers in the United States now argue that educational equity is not merely a democratic ideal but a practical necessity for building a healthy and productive society that can compete in a global economy.

American education could benefit from tackling inequality as the Finns did. We could make teaching a more highly paid and competitive profession that would attract the best-qualified college graduates. There is also a need for us to make an about-face on the practice of simply throwing more instructional time and more homework at underperforming students in hopes of getting them to learn more. More instructional time with a teacher who has already spent long hours in the classroom does not improve student performance, nor does piling on extra hours of homework. Giving an underperforming student one or more hours a day with a superior teacher who spends fewer hours in the classroom and is energized by having time for professional development is what really inspires a child to learn more.

The excessive homework that American students face each day, starting as early as first or second grade, does not necessarily enhance their learning. In my clinical experience, I have noticed that children who spend long hours doing homework are more likely to feel anxious and frustrated, as are their families, than to learn at a faster pace. Here again, we can benefit from Finland's educational philosophy of "less is more." According to international surveys, Finland's students have the lightest load of homework in the world, and Finnish parents do not need to scramble to find tutors or test preparation programs for their kids. Even in high school Finnish students don't have private tutoring or additional instruction outside of what is offered by their school.

American schools not only favor well-to-do students, they are also becoming increasingly slanted toward the learning style of girls. Simply being a boy in the United States carries an increased risk of being diagnosed with ADHD. In fact, boys are more than twice as likely as girls to be diagnosed with ADHD. Some experts have suggested that the higher rate of ADHD diagnoses in boys indicates that American schools are now geared to girls. A boy who does not behave like a quiet compliant girl in the classroom is seen as deviating from the norm. And in our medicalized society, deviating from the norm tends to be interpreted to mean there is something "biologically wrong" with the child.

Boys have more energy, curiosity, and impulsiveness than girls. When schools cut down on recess and physical education, they make school a less welcoming environment for boys. And the trend is not limited to the United States. The British Parliament set up a Boys' Reading Commission to address boys' underachievement. In its report, issued in

2012, the commission found that in 76 percent of UK schools, boys did not do as well in reading as girls. Girls spent more time reading than boys and enjoyed it more. The commission concluded that boys' underachievement was not due to biological differences or ADHD, but rather to social factors. British teachers are mainly women and tend to have limited knowledge of books that are interesting to boys. And because of the smaller number of male teachers, boys did not have enough role models of men reading for pleasure and learning.

The Ritalin Generation

Author Bronwen Hruska observed, in a 2012 *New York Times* opinion piece called "Raising the Ritalin Generation," that when her ADHD-diagnosed son, Will, was in fifth grade, he had a teacher who "didn't seem to know what to do with boys at all." Even though Will had been taking Ritalin since third grade, he couldn't settle down in his fifth-grade classroom. Will's psychiatrist upped the dosage, then switched medications twice, but nothing improved the situation. Hruska began to believe the pills had never helped Will at all. In fourth grade, he had had a teacher who liked him. She did not think he was annoying, just that he needed extra attention and support. The change in Will's social environment in fifth grade made all the difference in how comfortable he felt in the classroom and therefore how he behaved.

Hruska contended that our schools are narrowing the range of what is "normal" and observed that we are drugging kids who used to be considered normal but don't fit into the new standards. In my experience these worrisome comments ring true. We are raising the level of competition in our schools with performance-enhancing drugs such as Adderall and Ritalin. There is no room in today's classrooms for horsing around to break up the stress. We're also teaching our children to face the challenges they will encounter in adolescence and adulthood by taking mental steroids instead of learning how to control their behavior and develop the emotional skills necessary to cope with life's challenges.

Today in the United States, a student with above-average grades and compliant behavior is considered "mentally healthy," whereas a kid who goofs off at school and doesn't stand out academically is diagnosed with a *DSM-5* mental disorder. In our pharmed culture, mischievous boys like Tom Sawyer and Huck Finn would not be seen as active, adventure-loving kids who skipped school now and then because they were bored in a classroom that offered them little of interest. Society today would label them "mentally disabled" and give them drugs to make them behave like "normal" children.

Some children, especially high-energy though otherwise normal boys, appear to have ADHD only in certain settings. Our society's new standard of the "normal" schoolchild is too often blind to the influence of teachers. Many parents have found that while their child seems to have symptoms of ADHD with one teacher, when they change the child's classroom, put him in a different school, or even turn to homeschooling, the child does just fine—no diagnosis or medication needed.

Teachers are not the whole story, of course. Boys and girls need the opportunity for physical activity and engagement with nature. They need play that is not goal-oriented and that allows them to indulge their inquisitiveness and imagination. With most mothers and fathers at work all day, worries about child safety have escalated to the point that many children spend their after-school hours playing computer games or watching TV instead of playing ball or bicycling around the neighborhood with other kids. Children today spend half as much time outdoors as their parents did. Yet outdoor play improves children's health. Active play increases bone strength and lowers blood pressure and improves a child's ability to concentrate.

I grew up in south Florida, and I swam or biked with my friends after school until our mothers called us in for dinner. Spending free time outdoors on our own inspired our creativity and boosted our curiosity. Famed psychologist Alice Miller reminds us that aimless play is critically important because it helps children develop an authentic self. In play, children are the sole rulers of their small kingdoms. When they are deprived of opportunities for self-directed creative play, Miller says, they are likely to have problems. Even computer and video games are goal-oriented and are created by adults, not by children.

Research shows that more time for physical education and recess— healthy outlets for kids' energy—improves children's attention and concentration and their ability to stay on task. But many physical education programs have been defunded, and boys (as well as girls) are not getting the exercise they need for good mental and physical health. No wonder boys (and many girls) get fidgety in today's schools. The rationale for these cuts is that ebbing resources should be spent on core academic topics like math and science. But even learning core topics too often means just sitting in a classroom and listening to a teacher, instead of learning by doing—which includes physical activity. A Canadian study on improving boys' literacy recommends that classrooms use games, contests, and debates as learning tools—activities that appeal especially to boys' delight in competition.

Immaturity or ADHD?

There is also a strong argument for children to start school when they are older than five or six. This is especially important for boys, whose brains mature later than girls at this age. Malcolm Gladwell famously observed in his book *Outliers* that children who are among the oldest in their classrooms have a significant academic and social edge over their younger classmates. Most children begin school the September after their fifth birthday or even before they turn five if their school's cutoff date is later than September. Gladwell found that kids born between January and April—who are the oldest in the class—do better in school than their younger peers. Children who have summer or fall birthdays, and start school right after or before turning five, are at a disadvantage in achieving both athletic and academic success.

A 2010 study published in the *Journal of Health Economics* found that being born just before the kindergarten eligibility date increases a child's chances of receiving an ADHD diagnosis. Younger children are simply less mature than their classroom peers, and the study notes that "this behavior is misinterpreted as indicating that the child has ADHD." Shockingly, the researchers found that approximately 1.1 million American children received an inappropriate ADHD diagnosis and more than 800,000 were prescribed stimulant medications because of nothing more than their relative immaturity with respect to their older classmates. The study argues that diagnoses of ADHD are driven largely by subjective comparisons across children in the same grade in school.

Research from Britain similarly finds that a summer birthday can affect a child's academic achievement and also that the child is more likely to be diagnosed with a mental disorder—not only ADHD, but also autistic spectrum disorder and/or learning disabilities. Pulling together findings from studies of more than six thousand children, British researchers concluded that "children born in the months of May to August—the youngest in their year groups—were twice as likely to be identified as having 'special language and communication needs' than children born between September and December." The study took place in schools with a September cutoff date. The research took into account a number of factors, including economic status and race, along with month of birth. Teachers, the study noted, are inappropriately identifying children as having special educational needs when in reality they are merely younger than their classmates.

These results support findings of studies in Canada and Iceland. Researchers at the University of British Columbia found that kids born in December (the cutoff month for entering school) were "48 percent more likely to be diagnosed with ADHD and given medication, compared to children with January birthdays." The researchers also found that kids who take stimulants have slower growth rates and are at increased risk for sleep disruption and heart problems. They are also exposed to social stress, since teachers, parents, and peers may perceive them negatively throughout their school years. The Icelandic study, which tracked nearly twelve thousand children, found that those in the youngest third of their class were 50 percent more likely than their peers to be diagnosed with ADHD and medicated. According to this study, being younger affects children's academic performance all through their school years.

Childhood Adversity

Gender and age both affect a child's risk for being diagnosed with ADHD. But there are also more dire risk factors. Children who suffer severe family adversity or traumatic stress often develop behaviors such as impulsivity, hyperactivity, and inattentiveness. These experiences are known as ACEs (adverse childhood experiences) and may include emotional, sexual, or physical abuse or neglect, or living in a family situation that involves domestic violence, divorce, or substance abuse.

The landmark ACE study, sponsored by the Centers for Disease Control and Prevention in the 1990s, revealed that adverse childhood experiences, even among white upscale families, were far more prevalent than previously thought. This unexpected realization led neuroscientists to ask whether ACEs could go beyond behavioral effects and actually produce changes in children's brains. In 2010, a team of researchers at the University of Wisconsin found that indeed they could do just that. After querying more than four thousand adults about ACEs in their early lives, the researchers found that negative early experiences led to poorer mental and physical health, poorer school and work success, and lower socioeconomic status in adulthood. This indicates that prolonged stress early in life can have long-term effects by changing the circuitry of a child's brain.

How does this happen? Scientists found that over time elevated levels of stress hormones flood the brain and inhibit the prefrontal cortex, the part of the brain in which conscious learning takes place. Prolonged stress puts the brain into what scientists call a "fight, flight, or fright (freeze) mode," weakening the brain's other synaptic connections. This means that the social environment and the neurological map of the brain are connected and that children's brains, which are especially "plastic" or malleable, are influenced by experience. A child can have a neurological problem that is caused not by a genetic predisposition toward a "chemical imbalance," but by high levels of stress in his social environment. Modern neuroscience has thus closed the gap between nature and nurture. With respect to ADHD-type symptoms, those who insist that the problem is neurological and those who hold that the cause is environmental are both correct.

The ACE study inspired pediatricians in the United States to rethink their views about child development, giving more credence to the impact of environmental stressors. The authors of an article on the lifelong effects of childhood adversity and toxic stress, published in *Pediatrics* in 2012, suggest that it is time for a paradigm shift in pediatric medicine that gives environmental factors (nurture) more significance. They argue that the process of child development should no longer be viewed as primarily biological (nature) but as "nature dancing with nurture over time." From infancy through childhood, development is driven by an interaction between a child's genetic makeup and his social environment. As the new science of epigenetics is discovering, our early experiences get under our skins and into our brains, and they even impact the expression of our genomes.

Childhood Trauma or ADHD?

The ACE study heightened awareness, not only among pediatricians but also in the broader medical community, of how severe adverse experiences can affect a child's school performance and behavior. Research at Washington State University showed that ACE level was a powerful predictor for school attendance, behavior issues, and academic problems. Trauma researchers have known for a long time that children who have experienced traumatic stress at home have trouble controlling their emotions and impulses and focusing on their schoolwork. Trauma expert Bessel van der Kolk estimates that each year one million children in the United States experience abuse. The reactions to that abuse can take the form of inattention, impulsivity, and impaired executive function, which is the brain's ability to reason, problem-solve, plan, and stay on task. These reactions show that symptoms of childhood trauma are nearly identical to symptoms of ADHD. In one study, 67 percent of boys with histories of both physical and sexual abuse displayed symptoms that would qualify them for a diagnosis of ADHD.

The pediatricians who authored the *Pediatrics* article on childhood adversity emphasized the important policy implications of the ACE research, declaring that our education system has a social imperative to provide equal educational opportunities regardless of economic, racial, or ethnic status. To prepare our country's future workforce, the authors say, the conversation about improving the quality of early childhood education must involve more than educational objectives. It must also include investment in interventions that reduce adverse experiences in children's home environments. Such investments in all demographic groups "would generate even larger returns to the whole of society." Of course, as we have seen, adversity and extreme trauma are not the only factors that contribute to a diagnosis of ADHD. Middle- and upper-middle-class children are diagnosed as well. The doctors writing the article are addressing an often overlooked aspect of the ADHD epidemic.

Childhood adversity affects not only a child's preschool and later school performance but also his future mental and physical health. Intervening early with children at risk for adversity across all demographic sectors protects our whole society from the high costs of severe mental and physical health conditions that the child might have in adulthood. The authors of the *Pediatrics* article believe that risk factors that lead to demographic disparity in educational achievement and physical well-being "threaten our country's democratic ideals by undermining the national credo of equal opportunity." They urge the implementation of more effective strategies for addressing the disparities in child health and development that result from differences in social class, race, and ethnicity. These pediatricians have reached essentially the same conclusion that the Finnish government did in the 1970s when it charted a course toward educational equity.

Of course, pediatricians cannot meet all of a child's needs. Children must have a village of caring adults whom they can trust. When they do not feel secure and safe at home, society must enlist adults who can help provide that security. New research on the effects of trauma suggests that our schools need to evolve in order to meet the needs of each individual child. Instead of labeling traumatized children with ADHD and referring them for medication evaluations, schools are beginning to realize that having a good relationship with a supportive adult at school can mitigate the effects of traumatic stress on the child, and that it's more effective to create innovative interventions that help these kids right at the school.

A New Role for Schools

As a result of the ACE study and other research, schools are stepping up to the plate to play an increasingly supportive role for children who face adversity at home. Training workshops for teachers and school staff are helping personnel become sensitive to the powerful negative effects of extreme traumatic experiences at home, like the experiences in the ACE study. The programs look at the entirety of a child's school experience. They train not only teachers, school counselors, and school nurses but also cafeteria workers, playground monitors, office staff, custodians, and school bus drivers. Adults who work with children are learning to ask not "What's wrong with this child?" but rather "What happened to this child and how can I help?" Children who lack support from adults at home are benefiting from these relationships with adults at their schools. One typical intervention is providing children a safe, comfortable retreat at school, usually in the principal's office. Principals all over the country are inventing creative solutions to help kids feel safe and secure at school.

Otis Orchards Elementary School in Spokane, Washington, designates the first fifteen minutes of the school day a transitional time between home and school. During this "Opportunity to Interact with Students" Otis Orchards students are free to talk with their teacher, school counselor, or principal. Every morning, teachers greet students at the front door of the school and at the doors of every classroom. The kids know that they will have time to talk and express their feelings if they need to. The school principal, Suzanne Savall, often intervenes directly with her young charges. When a child comes to school crying or looking upset, Savall talks to him and allows him to express his feelings until he feels calm and comfortable enough to return to the classroom.

One day a second grader came to school in tears. As the principal questioned him gently, she learned he had witnessed his father hitting his mother and being taken away by the police. The principal brought the boy into her office, wrapped him in a blanket, and let him listen to music on headphones. Every five minutes she checked in and asked if he wanted to talk. Finally, he confided that he was scared for his mother. Savall picked up her phone and called his mother, who was able to reassure her son that she would be fine. After the phone call, the boy drew in the sand of a rock garden the principal keeps on her desk. This calmed him, and he was soon able to return to his classroom. When Savall checked in with him in the afternoon, he was doing fine.

Savall also changed the way she deals with aggressive behavior on the playground. Previously, a child who hit a classmate or defied instructions had to stand against the wall and was not allowed to participate in recess. Now, if it's the first time the child has been aggressive or oppositional, the teacher in charge asks him to apologize and promise not to do it again. She doesn't call the child's parents and request they pick him up from school. If it happens again, the child knows he will get five days on the wall and the principal will call his parents. The strategy is working well—only one child out of twenty-five repeated the aggressive behavior. Incidents of aggressive behavior—pushing, hitting, physical aggression—dropped from 83 to 13 during January to April 2013 compared with the same time period in the previous year. Otis also earned the School of Distinction Award for being in the top 5 percent of state schools in improvement of overall reading and math test scores.

Tackling Childhood Adversity

Some state legislatures are currently considering legislation that would require all schools in the state to draw on trauma research to create supportive environments. Vermont is the first state to consider a bill that calls for integrating screening for ACEs in health services. The Vermont bill even suggests incorporating research on ACEs into the curricula of medical schools and into continuing education programs for health professionals.

On June 17, 2014, the California Assembly Health Committee approved, by a vote of 16–0, a resolution to encourage statewide policies to reduce children's exposure to adverse childhood experiences. The California bill ACR 155 (which stands for "Assembly Concurrent Resolution 155") makes the case for state policies to "consider the concepts of toxic stress, early adversity, and buffering relationships" and to note "the role of early intervention and investment in early childhood years." The bill specifies that "the state's policies should consider the principles of brain development, the intimate connection between mental and physical health, the concepts of toxic stress, adverse childhood experiences, buffering relationships, and the roles of early intervention and investment in children."

Washington State has launched an innovative "compassionate school" program to help traumatized children feel safe at school. As more research emerges on how trauma affects children's brains and impacts their learning and behavior, other states and communities are creating "trauma sensitive" schools. With innovative programs in place, there is little doubt that the number of children diagnosed with ADHD in these schools will decline.

Individual school districts are responding to ACE research as well. In 2013, the Los Angeles Unified School District banned suspensions for defiance. Schools are trying to help troubled students before their reactions to trauma at home trigger a punitive response from teachers. After their parents have given permission, students are given an ACE questionnaire with questions like: "Have you been slapped, punched, or hit by someone?" and "Has anyone close to you died?" A student who has experienced trauma meets individually and in small groups with a social worker at the school. If they are willing, the child's parents meet with the social worker as well and are often referred for counseling at a mental health clinic that specializes in child trauma. One Los Angeles elementary school developed a support team, consisting of the principal, a social worker, teachers, coaches, and administrators, that meets regularly to help 25 percent of the school's students, who have been flagged for behavior, attendance, or academic concerns.

Someone Would Have Told Me in Medical School

Training school personnel to recognize the effects of ACEs and give traumatized kids extra help cannot alone solve the problem of traumatized children. Education in medical schools must change as well. Pediatricians, child psychiatrists, and family physicians must be taught about how adverse family experiences affect children and how trauma mimics the symptoms of what doctors now think of as ADHD. Dr. Vincent Felitti, coauthor of the ACE study, conducted an earlier study on obesity in 1980 at Kaiser Permanente. While talking to the participants of the obesity study, he asked them questions about their childhoods. He was shocked to find that one person after another had experienced trauma early in life. Though the subject of the study was obesity, Felitti was struck by the revelation that early childhood trauma was so widespread. After concluding the obesity study, Felitti said in an interview, "This can't be true. People would know if that were true. Someone would have told me in medical school." Tragically, they didn't; childhood trauma is not on the curriculum in most medical training.

There are indications that times are changing. In a surprising step forward, two widely cited *Pediatrics* articles, published in 2011 and 2012, addressed the issue of toxic stress. The authors warned that toxic stress early in life is the most prevalent peril to children and they urged pediatricians to recognize that stress can produce physiological effects on the child's brain. "The reduction of toxic stress in young children ought to be a high priority for medicine as a whole and for pediatrics in particular," they wrote. This is a good start. However, in their everyday practice, not enough pediatricians have yet made the connection between "toxic stress" and behavior that may be misdiagnosed as ADHD. If they had, the rate of ADHD would not still be climbing.

Using medication to suppress the life story of a child who is suffering from trauma subjects him to yet another form of maltreatment. Just as physicians systematically rule out various causes when they diagnose a childhood illness, pediatricians and psychiatrists should be required to rule out trauma before diagnosing a child with ADHD or other mental disorder. This means that physicians must interact with schools, children's services, and other social agencies. This is part of the new "ecological" paradigm of pediatric care urged by the pediatricians who authored the *Pediatrics* articles on childhood adversity and toxic stress.

Kyle

In my experience, a stressful event does not have to qualify officially as an ACE in order to trigger behaviors associated with ADHD. Parents' arguments and threats of divorce, a parent's depression, even a parent yelling at a child too often can cause that child to become irritable, impulsive, or aggressive. This is what happened with a five-year-old boy named Kyle.

Kyle's parents, Nora and Alan, called me because their son had become aggressive in kindergarten. Although their pediatrician had not yet made a diagnosis of ADHD, she recommended they try giving Kyle Adderall XR, which she thought might calm him down. But Nora and Alan were reluctant to give Kyle medication; they had heard about side effects and they knew about kids who wound up staying on drugs for years.

When I greeted Alan and Nora in my waiting room, they both looked worried and strained. As we talked in my office, it quickly became clear that they were facing serious challenges. A year earlier, Alan had been laid off from his job as a fund-raiser at an animal-rights organization. Like many nonprofits, his had suffered severe funding cuts, and they reluctantly had to let several employees go. Alan loved his job and was good at it. He was disappointed to lose it, but at first he was able to keep his spirits up, confident that he would find another position, if not in the fund-raising sphere then in some related field.

Alan called and e-mailed everyone he knew; he answered every ad and consulted headhunters and employment agencies. But after two months of futile searching he fell into a depression. This was a new experience for Alan, who was not prone to depression and usually managed stress well. He tried to keep up his physical regime, running each morning and swimming at the local YMCA, but more and more he found himself low in energy and unmotivated. Sleepless nights made everything worse. He did finally find a job in sales at an office supply store, at a much lower salary than he had had before. He continued to pursue possibilities in fund-raising, but his mood darkened as opportunities didn't pan out.

At the same time, Nora's job at a financial services company was becoming increasingly stressful and insecure. They recently had a second round of layoffs, and everyone felt the pressure of having to do more than their share of the work. Fearing that she, too, would be fired, Nora was putting out feelers for another job, but nothing had developed.

"We are always worried about money," Nora told me. "I think we've both become short-tempered—it's so tough for us. The school is giving us a hard time about Kyle's hitting other kids in the classroom, and lately he's been having tantrums at home. He throws toys around and breaks things. And sometimes, even though we don't mean to, we both end up yelling at Kyle. He just doesn't let up, and we give him what he wants because we don't have the energy to keep arguing. We know we shouldn't." Alan nodded his head in agreement, but I had a sense that his view of the situation was not quite the same as Nora's.

In our second session, I learned that although Alan loves Kyle dearly, he never wanted to have children. He was convinced that the torment they were going through with Kyle was his wife's fault because she talked him into having a child. They didn't agree about discipline. Nora thought they should have strict rules for Kyle about misbehavior and immediate consequences such as time-outs or taking away privileges.

Alan preferred a more collaborative and democratic approach to discipline, with Kyle taking part in the process. Alan's parents had been authoritative, spanking him and his brother when they misbehaved. Alan wanted to raise his son differently. Yes, he admitted, he yelled at Kyle—they both did—especially when they felt pushed too far. "We have never spanked him, though," Alan assured me.

I was glad to hear that, but I also knew that according to the latest research, parents' yelling can lead to aggressive behavior in kids almost as much as spanking. Psychologists at the University of Michigan and the University of Pittsburgh found that even a close, loving relationship with parents cannot protect kids against the harm caused by harsh yelling. It turned out that spending more time talking with the child about good behavior, and taking away privileges such as video games or television, were more effective and less damaging strategies than yelling at a child.

When had Kyle started misbehaving? I asked Nora and Alan. He had always been an active child, they told me, but in the months since Alan lost his job, he had become out of control. "When Kyle gets angry," Nora said, with tears in her eyes, "he kicks, hits, and bites other children. At home, when he doesn't get what he wants, such as candy or ice cream, he falls into rages. He knocks pictures off tables, turns over chairs; he once made a deep gash on his bureau with Alan's screwdriver." As I listened to Nora and Alan, the image of an *enfant roi*, or "child king," came to mind. Kyle had indeed become a tyrant, ruling the household with his rage.

Alan picked up the story. He told me Kyle's teacher said that even though Kyle is bright, he doesn't always pay attention in class. The only way he will complete a work sheet is if she sits next to him and gives him one-on-one attention. If the teacher or an aide is not available, Kyle daydreams or wanders around the classroom. I was not surprised to learn that Kyle was among the youngest in his class, having just turned five in July.

Kyle's teacher had been patient with him and hoped he would grow out of his inattentiveness. She was aware that Alan had been laid off, and she knew that a loss like this can affect a child. Now she was worried that Kyle would not be able to focus well enough to move on to first grade. She arranged for Kyle to meet with the school counselor once a week in a small group. At first, the group sessions seemed to help Kyle's moods, but the improvement in his behavior did not last.

One day, after hitting another boy on the school playground, Kyle ran away and tried to climb the playground fence. When a teacher attempted to get him down, Kyle bit her. Eventually, he did climb down and a special education teacher walked with him to the principal's office. The principal allowed Kyle to sit in a soft cushiony chair while he cooled down. She encouraged him to talk about what was troubling him, and eventually Kyle was able to express his frustrations. He said that he wished his father wasn't so sad and that his parents didn't yell at him so much. The next day, the principal met with Nora and Alan and suggested that they seek family therapy. That's when they contacted me.

Although Kyle was not abused or neglected, his parents' inability to discipline him effectively, their yelling, and his father's depression were upsetting him and causing him to act out. Sometimes when a parent is depressed, a child will misbehave just to get a reaction. In a child's mind, getting negative attention from a depressed parent is better than no attention. I would have to help Alan look for ways to become less depressed, and then I would need to help him and Nora find a method of discipline that worked for them. Alan's depression was more situational than chronic. I encouraged him to continue looking for an opening in nonprofits, and in the meantime to enhance his résumé with more education. I pointed out that he had many years of experience and excellent references. Surely he would find a good job before long.

By this time Alan had become so dispirited that he had practically given up running and barely made it to the gym for a weekly swim. I knew that more exercise would improve his mood, so I urged him to start running again. He didn't have to be at work until nine o'clock, so he had time to run a couple of miles in the morning before dropping Kyle off at school at eight thirty. The running helped Alan feel better about himself.

I also worked out an iron-clad agreement about discipline on which both Alan and Nora agreed. They knew it wouldn't be easy, but they realized they had to do something. We wrote down clear rules and consequences in a language that a five-year-old could understand. They decided on the "count to 3" strategy, which had been effective with my own children. When they said "1" it was a warning, "2" was getting close to a time-out, and if they had to count to "3" Kyle got an automatic and immediate time-out in his room. If necessary, Alan would physically restrain Kyle with a bear hug to put him in his room and keep him there. They were determined not to yell or to give in to Kyle's tantrums.

A behavioral plan like this needs to include positive reinforcement. At my suggestion, Nora and Alan made a star chart to track Kyle's good behavior. When he had a full day without time-outs at school or at home, his parents gave him a gold star. At the end of the week, four gold stars earned him a new toy or a trip to his favorite pizzeria. Kyle's teacher started a behavioral plan in the classroom as well. She created a similar star chart for all the children in the class and made Kyle the star monitor. Kyle felt proud of his new responsibility.

With consistent rules for behavior and his parents not yelling at him, Kyle slowly began to behave better at home and at school. Once, when a classmate hit him, Kyle told his teacher instead of hitting the boy back. His teacher praised him and gave him a gold star for improvement. Heartened by his teacher's praise and the gold stars, Kyle started applying himself more in the classroom. After a month, he was no longer inattentive. His teacher sent home notes of praise instead of the incident reports that his parents had dreaded so much. Sure Kyle could still be rambunctious at times. What five-year-old boy isn't? But he was no longer aggressive. Nora and Alan worked very hard to calmly and consistently give Kyle consequences for misbehavior, and the changes in their son more than repaid their efforts. After four months, they no longer needed to come to therapy except for an occasional "tune-up."

Because mainstream child psychiatry and pediatrics see childhood problems as biological disorders with genetic and/or chemical causes, Kyle easily could have been mislabeled with ADHD and given stimulants to control his symptoms. But the cause of Kyle's problems was not a genetic predisposition to behave badly and fail, but his environment. Although Kyle's brain might look different from the brain of a child from a calm home, the key to changing his brain was not chemical intervention but family and school intervention. Both Kyle's principal and teacher recognized Kyle's misbehavior not as deserving of punishment but rather as deserving of kindness and understanding.

The Increase of ADHD with "No Child Left Behind"

As we have seen, some schools are reinventing themselves to support children who suffer adverse experiences, just as the principal of Kyle's school knew to comfort and question him rather than to mete out punishment. We can only hope this trend will expand to include more school districts all over the United States. Paradoxically, however, the dominant paradigm of education in this country has actually led to rising rates of ADHD. In the four years after George W. Bush signed the No Child Left Behind Act into law in 2002, the nationwide rate of ADHD diagnoses increased 22 percent.

Why should this be so? The answer lies in the fact that the law tied financial rewards for schools to standardized test performance. Having more children diagnosed with ADHD was a boon to school districts that were lagging behind in test scores. First, scores for children diagnosed with ADHD could be omitted from the school's reported test scores. Second, children with the diagnosis got special accommodation, including extra time for taking standardized tests. Extra time, plus stimulant medication, which is a short-term performance enhancer, could very well raise kids' test scores, in which case the school could decide to include them with the rest of its scores. As a result, failing schools soon experienced a windfall of ADHD diagnoses.

This growth was already happening at the state level before No Child Left Behind. Some states had enacted laws that tied financial rewards to improved test performance, and ADHD diagnoses were exploding in poor-performing districts. For example, in 1997, 15.6 percent of North Carolina's children had an ADHD diagnosis. In California, the percentage that year was 6.2. North Carolina was one of the first states to link school financing to standardized test scores. California was one of the last.

Preschools Are for Play

Up to now, we have been talking about school-age children, but as the national conversation in the United States focuses more and more on providing preschool education for all children, new perils come to the fore. At the very least, we must take care to avoid high stakes testing for preschoolers. When school performance is measured by test scores, pressure to show success in state and federally funded preschools could lead to a rise in ADHD diagnoses. Since a child in the United States may now be diagnosed and medicated for ADHD as young as age four or even three, the ADHD epidemic would engulf even larger numbers of preschool children.

Preschool should be a time for play, imagination, and creativity. Children need to be able to bounce around, dance, sing, dress up in costumes, paint, and discover their interests. It also should be a time when children who are having behavior problems are evaluated and given individual attention. In Finland, as a matter of course, possible developmental deficits are evaluated even before children enter school, and those who are found to have learning or emotional difficulties receive special support from teachers and counselors. This approach prevents students from slipping behind instead of repairing their problems after they occur.

As we consider the policy for making preschools available to more children in the United States, which is still in the planning stages, we might well learn from Finland's practice of early intervention. This is especially important since the cost to society of prevention is always less than the cost of cure. The American Academy of Pediatrics can help in this effort by promoting increased awareness of the psychosocial causes of children's problems and by reevaluating its policy on diagnosing and drugging four-year-old children with ADHD. A study published in *Pediatrics* in 2013 found that parent-training classes are more effective than methylphenidate for treatment of preschoolers at risk for ADHD. The parent behavior training interventions were "designed to help parents manage their child's problem behaviors with more effective discipline strategies by using rewards and non-punitive consequences. An important aspect of each is to promote a positive relationship between parent and child."

Head Start Trauma Smart

An ACE-informed program called Head Start Trauma Smart already serves three thousand preschool-age children in Kansas and Missouri. More than 50 percent of the children in the program have experienced three or more ACEs. Students receive individual therapy through the program, but Head Start Trauma Smart also trains preschool staff to respond skillfully to the needs of traumatized kids. One school bus driver said that the trauma training has changed the way she deals with preschoolers. Instead of getting angry or impatient when her young passengers act out, she gives them hugs and reassurances. Although still in its early stages, the program has already been successful. Attention deficit problems and hyperactive behavior have decreased, and children who would have been labeled with ADHD have moved into a "normal" range of behavior for their age. A similar program for pre-schoolers in Washington State, called Safe Start, has also had promising results.

Nutrition is another important influence on children's mental and physical health. In the next chapter I look at how diet plays a role in children's behaviors and how dietary changes can help some children overcome behavioral and attention problems.

SEVEN

Let Food Be Thy Medicine

> Let me see if Philip can be a little gen-
> tleman; Let me see if he is able to sit
> still for once at table.
>
> • HEINRICH HOFFMANN

You don't usually allow your daughter to eat sweets, but once in a while you indulge her with a bag of M&M's, the most popular candy in the world. Does it make any difference if you purchase this treat in New York or London, in Kansas City or Paris? If, like most people, you said no, you would be wrong.

In fact, Mars, the giant food company based in McLean, Virginia, that makes M&M's, uses different ingredients in the United States and in Europe. For the M&M's they sell in the United States, they use artificial food dyes made from petroleum, including Red #40, Yellow #5 and #6, and Blue #1 and #2. These dyes give the candies their enticing fluorescent colors, but the M&M's Mars sells in Europe get their rainbow hues from dyes extracted from natural foods—for example, beets for red, carrots for orange, and saffron for yellow. To understand why the company has different formulas for different continents, we have to go back to the 1970s.

Food Allergies

In 1973, pediatrician and allergist Benjamin Feingold, chief of the allergy department at the Kaiser Permanente Medical Center in San Francisco, had a patient who suffered from severe swelling of her face. Searching for a way to relieve her symptom, he decided to try putting her on the Kaiser Permanente (abbreviated as K-P) diet. Feingold had developed this diet in the 1960s based on his own research and the research of Dr. Stephen Lockey of the Mayo Clinic. The diet was originally intended for treatment of skin conditions and asthma related to sensitivity to aspirin and other products containing an acid called salicylate. The K-P diet eliminated all artificial colors, preservatives, and flavorings, aspirin, and foods that contained salicylates, such as almonds, oranges, raspberries, apples, cherries, grapes, peaches, strawberries, cucumbers, plums, and tomatoes.

To Feingold's surprise, his patient's facial swelling disappeared almost immediately. He also observed improvement in her psychological problems. She had been seeing a therapist for two years because she was feeling hostility toward her husband, her friends, and her co-workers, but the therapy had hardly helped at all. After less than two weeks on the K-P diet, those negative feelings were clearly abating. The chief of psychiatry at the medical center was so amazed by this change that he called Feingold to ask what he had done for this patient to experience such dramatic results. When Feingold talked with her, she told him that on the K-P diet she felt she could completely control her behavior and her mood, but when she broke the diet and ate foods that contained artificial colors or salicylates, both her disturbed behavior pattern and her facial swelling recurred.

Alerted to a possible link between food additives and behavior, Feingold began observing children who came to the allergy department for various types of allergic reactions, such as nasal or skin conditions. As it happened, these children also exhibited behavior problems or hyperactivity, which at that time was called "hyperkinesis." Feingold prescribed the K-P diet for these children, and almost immediately both their allergic reactions and their hyperkinesis disappeared. To confirm these observations, he arranged for children whose primary complaint was hyperkinesis to be put on the K-P diet. The results supported Feingold's earlier observations: After only a few days on the diet the children calmed down so much and were so much more attentive to schoolwork and responsive to parents and teachers that those who were taking behavior-modifying drugs such as Ritalin could discontinue the drugs. When teachers rated the kids on a quarterly or semester basis, children on the diet who had been having difficulties at school showed a marked improvement in both their behavior and academic achievement.

Although 40 to 50 percent of the children in Feingold's study responded positively to the diet with a decrease in hyperactivity, he was not able to predict the response of any particular child. He therefore postulated that the reactions were akin to allergic reactions. Some kids were "allergic" to the artificial dyes and/or additives, and other kids were not.

Feinberg had prestigious credentials, both as an allergist and a pediatrician. He had spent a year in Vienna working under the supervision of Professor Clemens von Pirquet, who first coined the word "allergy." For six years, Feingold was chief of pediatrics at Cedars of Lebanon Hospital in Los Angeles. At Kaiser, he was chief of the allergy department as well as chairman of its central research committee. He also had written a well-respected textbook on pediatric allergy. After he presented his research at the 1973 meeting of the American Medical Association, he became a target of criticism, from both his fellow doctors and the packaged-food industry. Doctors criticized him for his reliance on clinical observations instead of conducting controlled studies. The AMA made a decision to prevent Feingold's ideas from being published in the *Journal of the American Medical Association.* However, he continued to publish his ideas in less renowned medical journals, such as *Ecology of Disease* and *Delaware Medical Journal.*

Interestingly, many doctors criticized Feingold not only because they found fault with his research but also because the results posed an enormous inconvenience to children and their families. Such an exacting diet would be difficult to carry out, his critics alleged, and might cause the child social isolation and even nutritional deficiencies.

Despite the flood of criticism leveled at Feingold, two subsequent studies confirmed his findings. One study was conducted at the University of Pittsburgh in 1976. The second was conducted in 1978 by the Food Research Institute at the University of Wisconsin. As in Feingold's research, not all children in these studies responded favorably to the diet, but 30 to 50 percent of them did and that was sufficient to make the results significant.

In November 1977, Feingold gave a talk at a meeting of the American Academy of Pediatrics about the effect of artificial food colorings on hyperkinesis in children. He presented a case of one of his patients, a seven-year-old boy who had extreme hyperkinesis, a case that the American Medical Association had refused to publish. At home, the boy stomped around, kicked the walls, and even charged oncoming cars on his bicycle. At school his behavior was so unruly that he had trouble learning. His family had consulted numerous experts—pediatricians, child psychiatrists, neurologists, and psychologists. Nothing helped until Feingold placed this boy on the K-P diet. After a few weeks the boy's hyperkinetic and disruptive behavior disappeared entirely; however, every time he strayed from the diet the behavior came back almost immediately.

In his presentation, Feingold addressed the question of the diet's inconvenience to a child's family. He found it difficult, he said, to believe that dietary intervention would entail greater family disruption than the many procedures recommended by the host of doctors they had consulted. In this talk, Feingold also raised the potentially explosive issue of doctors' "responsibility to industry," referring to the reactions of the food manufacturers. He was well aware of the significance of his findings for the food industry, he assured his audience, but in his view, a pediatrician's primary responsibility was to "the troubled children of the world."

Indeed, Feingold's work gave the packaged food industry plenty of cause for concern. He called for synthetic food additives and colorings to be regulated, just as pharmaceutical drugs were. The FDA, by and large, ignored Feingold's research on food dyes, although in 1976 it banned Red #2 after studies found that large doses could cause cancerous tumors in rats. The food industry replaced Red #2 with Red #40, which the FDA deemed to be safer. On the other side of the Atlantic Feingold's work would have a dramatically different impact. European food authorities became highly suspicious of synthetic food additives and closely watched further studies on artificial food dyes.

Following Feingold's work, a number of small studies in the United

States and abroad produced conflicting findings about the effects of artificial food dyes on hyperactivity in children. In 2004, a rigorous meta-analysis (survey of other studies) by researchers at Columbia, Harvard, and the New York State Psychiatric Institute found an "association" between the ingestion of artificial food dyes and hyperactivity. The team called for additional research and a broader discussion by society as to whether the "commercial rationale" for the use of artificial food colorings is justified.

The Southampton Study on Food Dyes

In 2007, inspired by Feingold, British researchers conducted a statistically rigorous study that drew wide attention and came to be known famously as the Southampton Study. Researchers at the University of Southampton in England had conducted an earlier study on the Isle of Wight that suggested artificial food dyes caused hyperactivity in three-year-old children. Now they sought to replicate these findings with a larger study commissioned by the British Food Standards Agency. They selected a cross-section of children from the general population, from both disadvantaged and affluent areas and from diverse socioeconomic and educational backgrounds. One group consisted of three-to-four-year-olds, the other group had eight-to-nine-year-olds. All the children behaved typically for their ages. None of them had been identified or diagnosed as having symptoms of hyperkinesis.

The study was double-blind and placebo-controlled, meaning that neither the moderators nor the subjects knew whether a particular subject received the active substance or a non-active substitute that mimicked the active substance in appearance and taste. Two mixes containing food colorings and the common preservative sodium benzoate were used. One mixture had the same quantity of artificial dyes as two bags of candy (2 ounces); the second mixture had dyes equivalent to four bags of candy (4 ounces). Three groups—teachers, parents, and trained observers—used several instruments to measure the children's behavior. Their observations correlated well. At the end of the six-week study, the researchers found an increase in the mean level of hyperactivity among typical children after they drank the mixture of artificial additives.

The Southampton Study was published in the respected British medical journal the *Lancet*. The conclusions, which confirmed Feingold's results, were incontrovertible. The research team concluded that "Artificial colours or a sodium benzoate preservative (or both) in the diet result in increased hyperactivity in 3-year-old and 8- and 9-year-old children in the general population." Not all children in the study were sensitive to the additives, but a significant number of them were. In the view of the Southampton team, removing artificial colorings from food would help the health of children. They were also careful to say that the sponsor of the study had no role in any aspect of the research. The researchers had no conflicts of interest.

When the study was completed, the British Food Standards Agency offered this advice to parents: "If a child shows signs of hyperactivity or Attention Deficit Hyperactivity Disorder (ADHD), then eliminating the colours used in the Southampton study from their diet might have some beneficial effects."

The EFSA (European Food Safety Authority) responded enthusiastically to the Southampton team's results. They wasted no time requiring that food companies place a warning label on foods containing the colorings the Southampton study had tested. The label would read: "May have an adverse effect on activity and attention in children."

The response of food companies to the Southampton Study was immediate and dramatic. Instead of agreeing to put the warning label on their products, food companies voluntarily switched to using dyes derived from plants. But they did this only for foods they sold in Europe. Even before the Southampton Study was published, when details of the study were leaked to the UK press, Asda, the UK branch of Walmart, voluntarily pledged to remove all artificial colors and flavorings from its products sold in Europe. A director at Asda said the company was acting because "mums and dads are becoming more and more concerned about what's in the food they buy." But Walmart did not change its policy in the United States, where mothers and fathers were presumably less concerned or at least less informed than British parents.

Coca-Cola Britain removed the additive sodium benzoate from products it sold in the UK. Kraft Foods UK also removed artificial colorings and flavorings from its food products aimed at kids, especially its popular macaroni and cheese products. Nestlé announced that the food products it distributed in Europe did not contain any of the additives investigated by the Southampton researchers. Instead, the company colored the food it sold in Europe with extracts of radish, lemon, red cabbage, and other vegetables and fruits, rather than the Yellow #6 or Red #40 it used in the United States.

While European agencies responded quickly to the Southampton Study, the United States Food and Drug Administration interpreted the findings differently. In 2010, the FDA issued an evaluation of the study that criticized every aspect of the research. It's worth noting that the evaluation included numerous comments by representatives of the food industry. A significant criticism was that the Southampton research did not offer data about the relative risks of individual dyes, making specific regulatory actions against individual colorings impossible. The Southampton team itself, meanwhile, had called for further research on individual dyes.

The FDA Disagrees

The FDA stated that food colorings merely affect a small group of people and need to be avoided by those select individuals only, as opposed to the entire public. The FDA thus concluded that the study had no utility. In 2011, it issued a statement conceding that certain "susceptible" children with attention-deficit/hyperactivity disorder and other problem behaviors could have their behavior exacerbated by exposure to synthetic food dyes. It added that the effects on children's behavior depended on the individual child's sensitivity to the additives and not on any inherent toxicity of the colorings. The FDA therefore left responsibility to individual food makers and to individual parents to decide whether to give children food products containing artificial additives. Their attitude was "Let the consumer beware." They did, however, throw the public one bone: They required that foods containing Yellow Dye #5 be clearly labeled because earlier studies had linked it to asthma.

In contrast to the FDA's unwillingness to take action on the issue, in 2012, China's Ministry of Health banned seventeen artificial food dyes and additives based on the findings of a panel of experts. One food safety expert expressed the panel's concern that "long-term consumption of such coloring could affect people's health, especially that of children."

At first, food manufacturers simply ignored the results of the South-ampton Study for products they sold in the United States. Switching to natural colorings was too expensive for them to bother with in the absence of FDA regulations requiring the switch. Artificial dyes were also brighter and more attractive to consumers, especially to children. But some influential Americans who had read the Southampton Study and the follow-up studies were moved to take action.

In a letter to Congress in 2000, Ohio State University professor of psychiatry L. Eugene Arnold made a plea for removing artificial food dyes in foods. He stated that "the only economic segment to suffer would be the dye manufacturers," and this cost should be weighed against solving a part of the ADHD problem. He argued that subsidiz-ing the dye industry's loss would be cheaper for taxpayers than the medical and educational costs of ADHD. In that same year, five mem-bers of Congress urged the FDA to state on its Web site that at least some ADHD children may benefit from dietary changes. The FDA re-fused to change its statement that studies failed to produce evidence that food colors could cause hyperactivity in some children. Nor was the American Academy of Pediatrics convinced that diet could influ-ence hyperactivity. The academy stated on its Web site that there was no scientific evidence that a change of diet could help children with hyperactivity.

Food companies labeled their products containing Yellow #5, as the FDA required, in as small a print size as possible and continued to mar-ket foods containing artificial colors and preservatives. According to the FDA's own data, food dye production enjoyed steady growth. Since 1955, food dye producers have come to rely on processed foods, such as soft drinks, breakfast cereals, candies, snack foods, baked goods, frozen desserts, and processed salad dressings. Food giants placed their bets on the likelihood that American parents were not familiar with the Southampton Study and would not take the time to scrutinize the fine print on a bag of Skittles, a box of macaroni and cheese, or a package of Pop-Tarts. And the food companies were right, at least for a few years.

The attack on Feingold's research by American physicians and by the food industry had a lasting effect. Even in 2011, four years after the Southampton Study's results appeared in the *Lancet*, the *New York Times* quoted pediatrician and ADHD specialist Lawrence Diller as claiming that the artificial food dye link to hyperactivity was merely an "urban legend" unsupported by scientific evidence. The Pharma-funded parent group CHADD also issued a statement dismissing the role of diet in treating attention and behavior problems. Children who might well have been helped by eliminating food dyes from their diets continued to be labeled with ADHD and treated with psychiatric drugs without dietary interventions even being tried.

Let the Consumer Beware!

In recent years, despite robust propaganda and heavy-handed marketing by the food and drug industries and Big Psychiatry, American consumers have started to wake up. As parents in the United States became informed about the effect of synthetic food additives on hyperactivity, they joined consumer advocacy groups such as the Center for Science in the Public Interest (CSPI) and started to put pressure on food companies. The CSPI started in a tiny borrowed office in 1971. Today, nine hundred thousand people subscribe to its *Nutrition Action Newsletter* and the center is supported primarily by subscribers to its newsletters and more than thirty well-known charitable foundations. It accepts no advertising, corporate funds, or government grants. In 2012, consumers achieved an important victory. General Mills removed artificial colors and flavors from its Trix yogurt products, which are pitched specifically to kids with the punchy slogan, "Trix are for kids." Trix yogurts now get their bright colors from vegetable juice, beta carotene, and turmeric extract.

Another victory came in 2013. Bowing to pressure from parents, food giant Kraft made a stunning decision. It announced it would voluntarily use natural spices instead of artificial dyes (Yellow #5 and #6) to give its popular macaroni and cheese products their distinctive glow-in-the-dark orange color. Following Kraft's lead, the cheese industry began to shift toward using annatto color (a natural derivative of achiote seeds) to replace Yellow #5.

Despite these decisions, however, and despite the fact that it has been banned in Europe, Yellow #5 dye is still one of the most commonly used food dyes in the United States. It is found in many products that appeal to kids, such as Frito-Lay SunChips, Lucky Charms breakfast cereal, Eggo waffles, and some Pop-Tarts products. Other dyes are found in yogurt, granola bars, chips of all sorts, candy, and even in children's medicines and vitamins. The popular Flintstones children's vitamins contain six artificial dyes, including Yellow #5. In 2013, the consumer protection group Change.org asked Mars to stop coloring M&M's and other candies it sells in the United States with petroleum-based artificial food dyes. Mars has yet to respond.

The medical community has taken a cautious stand. The Mayo Clinic states on its Web site that although there is no evidence that food additives actually cause ADHD in children, certain food colorings and preservatives may increase hyperactive behavior in *some* children. John E. Huxsahl, MD, author of the article on the Mayo Clinic's Web site, calls for more research on whether limiting processed foods could help prevent hyperactivity and other ADHD-like symptoms. He suggests that parents put their children on a diet that "limits sugary and processed foods and is rich in fruits; vegetables; grains; and healthy fats, such as omega-3 fatty acids found in fish, flaxseed, and other foods."

Healthy Diet, Healthy Children

My advice to parents is this: Even if you're not sure whether diet affects behavior, if your child tends to be hyperactive or inattentive, it will certainly do no harm to give him fresh, wholesome foods that don't contain artificial colorings or preservatives. In my experience, some parents actually do see improvement in their kids' behavior and school-work when they remove processed foods from their diets. Switching to foods with natural ingredients might be inconvenient and time-consuming at first, until you find healthier foods that fit your child's taste. But if your child is sensitive to artificial colors, flavors, and/or preservatives, the long-term benefits will certainly outweigh the short-term inconvenience. And it may even help your child without putting him on medication.

Prolonged situational stressors such as adverse childhood experiences or even inconsistent discipline and yelling affect a child's immune system and may make the child more vulnerable to synthetic food additives. With Kyle, the boy from the last chapter, an interesting connection emerged in my second therapy session with his parents. When I asked them if anything unusual had upset Kyle the day before the fence-climbing incident, they said he had gone to a friend's birthday party the evening before. The decorations on the birthday cake were brightly colored and there was plenty of candy for the children to eat. Although we certainly could not prove a connection between the birthday sweets and Kyle's unusually intense meltdown the following day, his parents felt that the two events were more than just a coincidence. Kyle's mother decided to be more careful about buying foods containing artificial colors and other additives and asked me the names of the specific dyes and preservatives to watch out for.

Another good choice is to add wild-caught fish or a fish oil supplement to your child's diet. Our grandparents' remedy of cod-liver oil to keep children healthy may well have some age-old wisdom in it. One study indicates that children with ADHD-type symptoms have low levels of certain essential fatty acids found mainly in fish. The University of Maryland Medical Center reports that in a clinical study of nearly one hundred boys, those with lower levels of omega-3 fatty acids had more learning and behavioral problems (such as temper tantrums and sleep disturbances) than boys with normal omega-3 fatty acid levels. Other studies suggest that supplementing a child's diet with omega-3 fatty acids can reduce ADHD-type symptoms at least in some children.

Some parents have told me that eliminating gluten from their child's diet produces a remarkable improvement in the child's ability to think and focus at school. Gluten is a protein found in wheat, barley, and rye. About 1 percent of Americans, or about two hundred thousand American children, have a sensitivity to gluten called celiac disease. The Mayo Clinic notes that the prevalence of celiac disease appears to be rising rapidly and has become a public health issue. One Mayo researcher speculates that changes in the way wheat is processed today as compared to fifty years ago might be responsible for the increase. Consumer groups in the United States and abroad have expressed concern about genetically modified wheat, which is grown with the help of toxic fertilizers and pesticides.

Some people are gluten intolerant but may not be diagnosed specifically with celiac disease. Gluten sensitivity often affects the gastrointestinal tract, but it can affect the central nervous system as well. In a 2004 article in *Pediatrics*, doctors found that celiac disease can produce learning disorders or ADHD-like symptoms in children. If your child's schoolwork improves when you remove gluten from her diet, you might consider taking her to your pediatrician or an allergist and having her tested for gluten intolerance or celiac disease.

And what about sugar? Although most parents observe that their children become out of control after eating sugary foods, there are surprisingly few good studies on the effects of sugar on kids' behavior. Whatever research has been done suggests that sugar may affect the behavior of a small number of children, but not as dramatically as parents tend to believe based on their own experience. Of course, even if studies indicate that refined sugars do not have a direct effect on kids' behavior, children should eat fewer sugary foods for good nutrition and to avoid obesity. And of course, many sugary processed foods such as processed desserts contain synthetic food dyes.

Some American restaurants are making small concessions by serving healthier, less sugary drinks to children. In 2014, McDonald's announced that it would no longer list soda on the kids' meal section of its menu board, and by 2015, soda will no longer be the default beverage in its popular Happy Meals. Restaurant chains Subway, Chipotle, Arby's, and Panera also have taken soda off their children's menus. But McDonald's still enhances the appearance of its brightly colored strawberry sundaes with Red #40 in the United States. In Britain, children can enjoy McDonald's strawberry sundaes colored only by the strawberries.

For those parents who eliminate artificial dyes and processed foods from their children's diets, there is no evidence to suggest that kids balk at the change. That said, the real key to getting children to enjoy eating fresh healthy foods is to get them accustomed to them at a young age. In France, which is famous for its love affair with food, children eat freshly prepared non-packaged foods from the time they are babies. In French day care centers as well as French homes, babies eat freshly pureed vegetables, fruits, and fish. For older children, lunches at preschools and schools preserve the tradition of giving children foods that are prepared from scratch without synthetic additives. French children have three or four courses at their school lunch. A typical lunch might consist of a first course of lettuce with vinaigrette dressing, a second course of grilled fish accompanied by a vegetable such as carrots or broccoli, a serving of cheese, and a fresh fruit or fruit tart for dessert. Of course, a freshly baked baguette (made without preservatives) accompanies the meal. And French children drink plain water with their meals both at school and at home instead of soda or sweetened juice.

In Finland, the first country in the world to serve free school lunches for all children, lunches and afternoon snacks teach kids good nutrition and healthy eating habits. Unlike American schoolchildren, Finnish children do not have Tater Tots, hot dogs, or warmed-up frozen pizza for lunch at school. Instead, they eat fresh vegetables, fish or meat, fruits and berries, whole-wheat bread, and skim or low-fat milk. Sugary drinks are banned from classrooms and dining halls.

Healthy Foods for Kids

In the United States, parents mainly have to go it alone to get their kids to eat wholesome foods. The school lunches of American children reflect the fast-food mentality of American culture. These lunches are often catered by junk food chain restaurants and are filled with artificial colors and flavorings. Parents can make sure their child eats a healthy meal in the middle of the day by packing their child's lunch. If your child is a picky eater, give him a say in what goes in his lunch box. Parents can offer a choice between wholesome alternatives of high-protein foods such as string cheese, hard-boiled eggs, and peanut butter or hummus sandwiches on whole-wheat bread. A sliced apple or pear, along with some trail mix or yogurt, make for a healthy dessert. These may be supplemented by a container of milk bought in the school cafeteria.

Ideally, a child's day should start with a hearty breakfast containing protein and omega-3 oils (from foods such as walnuts or fish or in a vitamin supplement). Some wholesome breakfast ideas that will help keep a child calm and focused are:

- Peanut butter (without added preservatives or sugar) on whole-wheat toast
- Scrambled eggs cooked in canola or olive oil
- French toast made from whole-wheat bread
- Unsweetened granola, muesli, or whole-grain cereal with milk and fruit
- Oatmeal with chopped walnuts, flaxseed, or Brazil nuts sprinkled on top
- Grilled cheese sandwich on whole-wheat bread

All of these should be accompanied by a glass of milk. Parents should consult their pediatrician to advise them on whether whole milk, low-fat milk, or nonfat milk is most suitable for their child.

What of the child who doesn't like to eat breakfast? I hear this from many children in my practice, and I've come to realize that early intervention is the best strategy. Get your children accustomed to eating a healthy breakfast from an early age so they don't question the routine later on. And parents can be good role models for their kids by eating a healthy breakfast that is rich in protein and low in sugar. Breakfast is also a good way to spend time with your kids. Sitting down for a wholesome breakfast not only engenders good eating habits but also allows you to talk with your child about the day ahead.

The Mayo Clinic Web site recommends nutrient-dense foods for children: protein, fruit, vegetables, grains, and dairy. For protein, it suggests fish, lean meat and poultry, eggs, peas, and unsalted nuts and seeds. Fruits and vegetables should be fresh if possible. If you allow your child to drink fruit juice, make sure it is 100 percent juice. The Mayo

Clinic also recommends whole grains such as whole-wheat bread, oatmeal, popcorn, or brown rice. Children need dairy products rich in calcium to build strong bones. This should be from fat-free or low-fat dairy products such as milk, unsweetened yogurt, and cheese. Getting children involved in planning meals, going grocery shopping, food preparation, and even growing vegetables in the backyard or in a community garden can get them interested in eating healthy foods. Most kids enjoy a trip to the local farmer's market with their parents, and farmer's markets are a good way to introduce them to new fruits and vegetables.

In the absence of regulatory constraints, American parents have more difficulty than their European counterparts in shielding their children from the marketing onslaughts of giant food companies. Hopefully, this will not be the case for much longer. American children and parents need the FDA to come forward and follow the example of its European counterparts. The FDA should stop acting on behalf of giant food corporations and restaurant chains and instead take responsibility for protecting our country's children against the callous practices of corporations that exploit them for profit.

A food diet is not the only thing that may affect a child's ability to focus and concentrate. In the next chapter, I'll look at how a child's media diet can affect hyperactivity and attention problems, and I'll show how some countries are taking action to protect their children from the unhealthy effects of inappropriate media.

EIGHT

Tweens, Teens, and Screens

> For every action, there is an equal and
> opposite reaction.
>
> • ISAAC NEWTON

In 1995, when my twin sons were twelve years old, they discovered the computer game Arctic MUD (multiuser dungeon), which had been developed in the early '90s. They played this exciting game on our old desktop computer, the only computer we had in those days, their chairs pulled close together so they could both see the screen and take turns on the keyboard. They also interacted with friends on the game, as well as with adults and kids all over the world. Arctic MUD was text only; there were no images of blood and gore. The objective of the game was to make one's character as powerful as possible by killing monsters and thereby collecting gold. Gold gave a character the power to ascend to higher levels, thirty levels in all. Spending time on the game wasn't interfering with our sons' schoolwork, their social lives, sports activities, or neighborhood paper route. They watched very little television (our tiny TV set was hardwired to PBS) and spent plenty of time reading books that interested them.

Their screen time on Arctic didn't pose any kind of problem as far as my husband and I could see. They were learning valuable keyboard skills and enjoying wholesome and challenging adventures. Arctic's interactive dimension made it more interesting than the simple puzzle-solving games they had played in the 1980s, like Tetris, Pac-Man, Mario Brothers, and the adventure game Myst, which our whole family had enjoyed for a time.

Then we began to notice that on weekends, after spending four to five hours playing Arctic, our sons became noticeably irritable and moody. My husband and I started to be concerned. So we asked the boys to limit their sessions to three hours at a stretch on weekends and one hour on weekdays. The boys thought this was reasonable, especially since they had plenty of other things to do. Once we limited the screen time, their moodiness and irritability disappeared. It was an interesting lesson about the effect of screens, even those without violent images, on kids' moods.

This was in the 1990s, when parenting teenagers seemed almost bucolic compared to today. It was before teens, tweens, and even younger children became seduced by an endless stream of electronic screens that disrupt their sleep, family life, and schoolwork in ways we could not have imagined back then. Our kids did not have cell phones they could tuck under their pillows at night in case one of their friends felt like calling or texting at 2:00 a.m. The Internet was in its infancy. The fastest dial-up bandwidth was 54 kilobits per second, while today home Internet speeds exceed 20 million bits per second and are available to even middle-class households. These days my four-year-old grandson connects to the Internet to watch cartoons on my son's smartphone. He can't watch them on television because his parents have chosen not to own a TV set.

When families came to my office in the 1990s, television was the only "screen" we discussed. If children were having attention problems at school, I recommended that parents limit younger children to one hour and older children to two hours a day of public television only. I also suggested that violent movies, videos, or television shows be entirely off-limits. In 1999, when the American Academy of Pediatrics recommended that children under two should have no screen time at all, I quoted this to parents. The rationale was that for healthy brain development kids that age need to interact and play with parents and other caregivers. They need real people to look at them and talk to them. Passively watching a TV screen does not fill this need.

I also advised parents not to put television sets in their children's rooms at any age. Instead they should encourage their kids to play outdoors, participate in an active sport, do craft projects, draw, paint, or read. Some parents thought my advice was unrealistic or even harsh, but as a therapist it just seemed like common sense. Based on my experience with my own children, I believe public television, in contrast to commercial programming, puts thought and care into the quality of its children's shows. And it does not interrupt the shows with commercials for fast foods and junk foods, which entice kids toward unhealthy eating habits and obesity. Studies had also shown that young children who watched educational programs on public television like *Sesame Street* and *Mr. Rogers' Neighborhood* performed better on academic tests.

Christakis's Research

Eventually, research backed up the advice I had been giving to parents. In 2004, a team led by the physician and sociologist Dimitri Christakis, of Seattle Children's Hospital at the University of Washington, conducted a study of one thousand children, the results of which appeared in *Pediatrics*. Christakis found a link between the amount of time toddlers spent in front of the TV and attention problems at age seven that could be diagnosed as ADHD. For every hour of television these young children watched each day, their risk of later having attention problems increased by 20 percent. The study concluded with this advice to parents: "Limiting your children's exposure to television as a medium during formative years of brain growth … may reduce children's subsequent risk of developing ADHD." Of course, biologically oriented experts criticized the study because it raised the issue of an environmental, not a biological, contributor to children's attention problems.

Since Pharma and Biological Psychiatry maintain that ADHD is essentially a "chemical imbalance" of genetic origin in the child's brain, a solution other than medication (i.e., less television) undermined their worldview. Christakis soon found himself under attack. It's important to note that he was not ignoring biological factors like genetics. He thought that if a child is predisposed, by genetics and/or social context factors, the probability of excessive television giving rise to attention problems is even higher. Thus limiting exposure to television could reduce attention problems even if there is a genetic component. It could promote healthy brain development and reduce the risk of a child developing ADHD. No psychiatric drugs required.

One particularly hostile critic of Christakis's study was psychologist Russell Barkley of the Medical University of South Carolina. Barkley is a recognized expert on ADHD and author of several best-selling books on the topic. He criticized the study on several grounds. For one, he said, it relied on parents' reports of how kids behaved and that parents were not qualified to diagnose ADHD. He also alleged that the investigators were biased toward blaming parents for their children's attention problems because parents allowed them to watch too much television. Barkley, a longtime promoter of the view that ADHD is a medical condition that a child is born with, has financial ties to Eli Lilly, the maker of the ADHD drug Strattera. From 2009 to 2012, he received $118,000 from Eli Lilly for consulting and speaking engagements, according to pharmaceutical company disclosures.

Big Bird or Spongebob?

In 2010, a large study at Iowa State University added video games to the mix of environmental factors that might be associated with children's attention problems. The team assessed 1,323 middle school children and 210 older adolescents over a period of thirteen months. They found that for both groups exposure to television and video games was associated with greater attention problems in the kids, as assessed by teachers. Moreover, children who engaged in more than two hours of daily screen time were at higher risk for developing attention problems. The researchers concluded that both video games and television were risk factors for attention difficulties.

The Iowa team observed that certain types of television programs and video games may pose more of a risk than others. They suggested, for example, that educational television may be safer than noneducational television "in terms of pacing or violent content or other features . . . which might account for such a difference." They noted that "there are many differences in features among video games, differences that may lead to differential effects on attention problems. As future research examines television and video games and their influence on attention problems, differences that are based on finer grained analyses of screen media features should be examined." The team concluded that slower-paced, educational, nonviolent content may be less likely to cause attention problems.

In 2011, researchers at the University of Virginia followed up on the Iowa study's recommendation for further research on the differences between educational and commercial television's effects. That is, they considered the *quality* and not just the *quantity* of television shows, and questioned whether attention problems were exacerbated if kids watched low-quality programs. The study, "The Immediate Impact of Different Types of Television on Young Children's Executive Function," appeared in *Pediatrics* in September 2011. The team divided sixty four-year-olds into three groups. Each group was put into a room and directed to do one of the following activities: draw with crayons, watch a PBS show called *Caillou* (about a little boy), or watch *SpongeBob SquarePants*, a fast-paced commercial TV show. After nine minutes of exposure to the given stimulus, the children took a series of tests that required focus, concentration, patience, working memory, and manipulation. Researchers were hoping to capture the "executive function" of a child's brain. Executive function refers to a set of cognitive skills like managing time, remembering details, switching focus, and integrating past experience with present tasks. ADHD is typically viewed as a deficit in executive function.

The results of this study were remarkably in tune with what common sense had been telling us for years. Children who watched cartoons on commercial television did significantly worse on the attention and memory testing than the children in the other two groups. There was no difference in performance between the educational TV (*Caillou*) group and the group that drew with crayons. The researchers concluded that shows on public television did not harm children's intellectual functioning.

Fast-Paced Cartoons

So what was it about the commercial cartoons that had a negative effect on the children's brains? The researchers concluded that the unnaturally fast pace of the cartoon sequences was overstimulating and stressful to the children's brains. The human-puppet interactions on *Sesame Street* and other PBS children's shows are naturally paced, whereas the *SpongeBob SquarePants* sequences are unnaturally rapid. Nickelodeon, the children's television station that produces *SpongeBob SquarePants*, criticized the study for its small size. Interestingly, Nickelodeon is also the corporate sponsor for an online gaming site called Addictinggames.com, which offers children fast-paced Internet games that often combine violence with sexual images.

In an editorial in the same issue of *Pediatrics* called "The Effects of Fast-Paced Cartoons," Christakis commented that although the study was small, the findings were nonetheless robust. He wrote, "Connecting fast-paced television viewing to deficits in executive function . . . has profound implications for children's cognitive and social development that need to be considered and reacted to." In other words, if kids spend too much time watching fast-paced images on television, they might develop symptoms of inattentiveness due not to any medical condition but to overstimulation of their brains.

Christakis emphasized that the University of Virginia study is important because it shows for the first time that the *quality* of TV shows is as important as the quantity of time children spend in front of the screen. "Television is both good and bad," says Christakis; "there are good programs and bad ones." And he goes on to say that it is not only the *content* of the show that makes it good or bad for children. It is the *form* or the way that content is presented. The real issue is whether the show is overstimulating for young brains. Christakis recommends not that kids be banished from all media but that parents steer kids to safe and educational media activities like PBS children's programs and educational computer games. In today's world, this is easier said than done. Indeed, it has become a major issue in my family therapy practice.

Brains on Games

In the 1990s, screens other than television, movies, and videos were rarely a concern in family therapy. Today, screens of all sorts play a central part in my work with families. It is estimated that young people in the United States spend between six and eight hours every day in front of screens, with electronic games trumping reading for enjoyment. Parents complain that they can't tear their kids away from video games when it is time to start their homework, that kids are texting when they are supposed to be sleeping, and that they stay up late at night on social media. Parents are also concerned that screen relationships are replacing real relationships for their kids and that texting is becoming obsessive. My teenage patients, for example, feel it is perfectly acceptable to receive and reply to texts during our therapy sessions.

In hindsight, my recommendation that parents limit children to one hour of public television a day seems almost quaint. Today's therapists spend increasing energy suggesting rules about the amount of time kids are allowed to spend on computer and video games, iPads, iPods, smartphones, Facebook, Twitter, and Instagram. Electronic technology seems to be tearing apart the very fabric of family life. Older kids are more attracted to spending time on screens with their "friends" than spending time with their families, and parents feel powerless to change this.

Heated public conversation about the effects of gaming on everything from bullying to school failure seems to have little impact. An entire segment of middle school and high school girls and boys identify themselves as "gamers." For a girl, being a gamer saves her from having to fit in with the "girlie girls" with whom she may have little in common. Boys tell me that being gamers gives them a group identity. Gamers tell me that they have trouble falling asleep at night, and that they only text their friends and play video games because they can't sleep. It's difficult to tell whether the reverse is actually the case and that kids have become so addicted to screens that they can't tear themselves away to rest their overstimulated brains.

Teenagers, though, are quick to defend their favorite games. One of my patients, a shy fourteen-year-old girl named Marianne, whose family recently moved to California from Michigan, has had a difficult time adjusting to a new high school. She spends after-school time in her room playing video games, despite her parents' entreaties for her to find activities that might help her make new friends. Marianne told me recently that a game called The World Ends with You helps her feel less lonely by allowing her to enter the imaginary worlds of other people. She likes a game called Persona for the same reasons. She says these games encourage her to be more social, at least on the screen, but so far her screen friendships have not translated into actual human relationships. Learning that Marianne was interested in animals and nature and planned to be a veterinarian, I encouraged her to get involved with an environmental group. I felt heartened recently when she attended a meeting of the local 4-H club and met a girl there who seemed nice. They were keeping in touch by texting. Marianne plans to continue going to 4-H meetings and is considering going on an overnight field trip with the club to Los Padres National Forest.

Other kids tell me that games like Minecraft stimulate their imaginations and creativity, and they can't understand why their parents object to them. In 2013, *New York Times* reporter Nick Bilton wrote an article examining the educational qualities of Minecraft and urged parents to calm down. Bilton gave examples of schools that use Minecraft to teach students skills. One school in Stockholm uses Minecraft to teach students "city planning, environmental issues, getting things done, and even how to plan for the future." In Australian schools, Minecraft helps students explore ancient worlds. However educational and enjoyable the game is, parents still need to moderate kids' time on electronic screens. One ten-year-old patient of mine developed facial tics from spending too much time playing games like Minecraft on his computer and smartphone. When his parents limited his screen time to one hour a day, the tics disappeared.

Teens seem to know they spend too much time gaming, but at the same time they rebel against the limits their parents try to place on them. Therapy sessions with teenagers and their parents often turn into heated negotiations about rules for using myriad media devices.

The American Academy of Pediatrics urges families to create a "media use plan" to help children make healthy media choices. A full list of its recommendations can be found on its Web site, healthychildren.org. Pediatricians in the AAP encourage parents to have a media curfew at bedtime and to take an active role in their children's experience by watching programs with them and discussing the values represented there. They suggest parents limit kids' screen time and require their children to go off the grid at mealtimes.

The AAP's recommendations have helped me defend my positions on screen time, which some parents see as downright draconian. In addition to asking parents to read and heed the AAP guidelines, I urge them to keep television sets turned off unless someone is watching a particular program. Having television on as "background" noise can be distracting to a child who is trying to focus on homework or reading for pleasure. I also advise that younger children watch shows that are specifically created for kids and avoid TV news shows, which often contain violent segments. One father, whose son had been referred to me for an ADHD evaluation, protested that watching the news when he came home from work helped him unwind. I suggested he record the show and watch it after his children went to bed. His wife proposed that he download the news to his phone and listen to it with headphones while he cleaned up after dinner. Feeling outnumbered, but taking it with good humor, the father agreed.

So pervasive is the perceived need for mobile phones in our society that one father actually balked when I suggested taking away his nine-year-old son's phone when he behaved disrespectfully toward his parents and teachers. The father believed that this would be tantamount to violating the child's "right to communicate," as if it were a violation of the First Amendment.

It should be no surprise, given the proliferation of overstimulating electronic media, that the diagnosis of ADHD is on the rise among American teenagers. However, there is a serious risk of mislabeling teens with ADHD when their inattentiveness and falling grades may be related to their media-infused lifestyle and resulting lack of sleep. This misdiagnosing was especially striking to me with a sixteen-year-old girl named Jeanette, whose family consulted me last February.

Jeanette

Rain was drumming on the roof and the windows of my waiting room when I greeted Jeanette and her parents. Jeanette looked younger than her sixteen years. She had olive skin and her shiny black hair was pulled back into a ponytail. She was dressed in jeans and a blue-and-gray UCLA Bruins sweatshirt. Jeanette's parents, Cheryl and John, were both teachers at a local university. They were visibly distressed as they walked from the waiting room into my office.

After introductions, I commented on the attractiveness of Jeanette's sweatshirt and asked if she was hoping to attend UCLA. She shook her head and told me her older brother was a sophomore there. "He's the whiz kid of the family," Jeanette said, her voice dripping with sarcasm. Cheryl grimaced. It was obviously not the first time she'd heard these words.

Up until last year, Cheryl told me, Jeanette had been a straight-A student. All her high school classes were either honors level or Advanced Placement (AP). But in the fall of her junior year, Jeanette seemed to lose her motivation. Her grades began to slip to Cs then to Ds, until finally she was close to failing two classes. Instead of studying, she stayed up late playing computer games and spending time on social media sites. She also showed signs of depression and anxiety—low energy, insomnia, and angst about seeing friends. After talking with Jeanette, their family doctor recommended that the family consult a psychiatrist. The psychiatrist prescribed the antidepressant Zoloft, but after six weeks it had had no effect. So he switched Jeanette to Lexapro, another antidepressant. He also prescribed the stimulant drug Adderall for what he thought was the ADHD keeping Jeanette from focusing on her schoolwork.

When I met the family, Jeanette had been on medication for four months, with little improvement in her mood or behavior. She could scarcely get out of bed in the morning. Fortunately, she was on the school tennis team and this motivated her to get to school eventually, although by now her tardiness had reached an almost unacceptable level. Even with the exercise she got at tennis, Jeanette complained of low energy. Finally, her psychiatrist had prescribed clozapine, a powerful antipsychotic drug typically used to treat bipolar disorder and schizophrenia in adults. Upset about their daughter taking such a strong drug, her parents started looking for alternatives. Their family doctor suggested they give family therapy a try and referred them to me.

Cheryl and John had been anxious about which Ivy League college Jeanette would get into. Now they worried she wouldn't graduate high school. As educators, they were embarrassed that their daughter wouldn't be going to a prestigious college. They found themselves avoiding parties and get-togethers with friends whose conversations centered on their children's college plans. I could see they were deeply hurt and confused about Jeanette's academic decline. They felt incompetent as parents, although they had always made a point of spending quality time with Jeanette and her brother. John had coached their tennis teams, and both parents had engaged with them intellectually, conducting lively conversation at the dinner table.

I wanted to know when Jeanette's depression had begun. With a yawn, Jeanette told me it started about six months ago. "What else was going on in the family at that time?" I asked her. Jeanette was silent for a moment. And then she said, "My parents were fighting almost every day. I could hear them from my room at night. I'm up late playing games on the computer. I hear everything." Then she started to cry. Finally, she said through her tears, "I heard my dad mention divorce. And my mom used that word, too." She stopped to compose herself. Then she looked me in the eyes and said in a small voice, almost a whisper, "I'm afraid that if I graduate high school and go away to college, my parents will get divorced." While Cheryl and John looked stunned at this revelation, Jeanette's answer did not surprise me in the least. Frequently a teenager or even a younger child will express her greatest fears about her parents in the very first therapy session. This happens so often that it seems to me kids are hoping therapy will actually help their parents.

Quickly changing the subject, John told me that on the advice of Jeanette's psychiatrist and her school counselor, Jeanette had dropped her AP and honors classes and was taking regular high school classes. Cheryl added they had stopped pressuring Jeanette about getting good grades and getting into an elite college. "We don't care anymore about college. We just want our happy daughter back." As she said this, a tear drifted down Cheryl's cheek. While John and Cheryl were talking, Jeanette continued to weep quietly.

As I often do when teenagers are involved, I had to conduct therapy with this family on two levels. I had to solve the family-system problem by meeting with the parents privately, and I had to resolve Jeanette's depression, attention problems, and anxiety by working with her alone. At first, Cheryl and John resisted my suggestion that their arguments might be affecting their daughter. They admitted that in the heat of anger they had occasionally mentioned divorce, but they had never seriously considered breaking up. However, they promised to keep their squabbles away from the house so that Jeanette could not overhear them.

One of their main issues was that Cheryl did not get along with John's mother who, she felt, had never accepted her as a daughter-in-law because she was African-American. I turned to John to get his opinion on this. He agreed with his wife. "It was hard for my mother at first," he said, "but after the children were born she was more accepting. Cheryl was very hurt about my mother's rejection in the early years of our marriage." "And your father?" I asked. "He was accepting of Cheryl from the beginning," John said. I looked at Cheryl and she nodded in agreement. "John's father has always been supportive."

"But what about Jeanette?" John asked. "Why is she getting such bad grades? Why is she staying up until two or three o'clock in the morning playing games on the Internet?" "She's too tired to get up for school," Cheryl added. They told me they were afraid to limit Jeanette's Internet time because the psychiatrist had advised them not to put any kind of pressure on her.

Strangely, though, when I met alone with Jeanette, she confessed that she worried she was "addicted" to the Internet. She knew she needed limits on her gaming because she wasn't getting enough sleep. But she found it impossible to cut back on her Internet sessions because without that distraction she started to worry about her parents or about what the other kids at school thought of her. The screen erased her worries. Late at night she sometimes texted with her classmate Kayla, whom she felt was the only friend she could talk to openly. In the mornings, Jeanette often felt sluggish and listless, as if she were addicted to a dangerous drug instead of a fun escape that had gotten the better of her. As addiction expert Dr. Gabor Maté has observed, addiction is located not in the addictive substance or activity but in the pain that people feel in their life circumstances. Addictions can spring from the inability to deal with the everyday stresses of a difficult life stage like adolescence.

In a family session, I was able to negotiate a compromise to help Jeanette. Her father would turn off the Internet in the house at 9:30 p.m. to help her overcome her addiction to late-night gaming. She would also turn in her smartphone to her parents at that time so she wouldn't be tempted to text or call Kayla. They would charge her phone overnight and give it back to her in the morning. In return, her parents would stop bugging her about starting her homework the minute she got home from school. On days when she didn't have tennis practice, Jeanette could play video games or do whatever she wanted until 6:00 p.m. Then they would remind her to start on her homework. Since she no longer had honors or AP classes, she rarely had more than an hour of homework.

Once the rules for Internet and phone were settled, I worked with Jeanette alone to help her with her fears. After our second meeting, she stopped weeping through the sessions. She told me that her parents were no longer quarreling. "At least in front of me," she added, with a twist of the side of her mouth that signaled her usual sarcasm. She was very aware of the ongoing tension between her mother and her grandmother, and she told me it worried her.

To help Jeanette control her anxiety, I asked her to spend a half hour each day in her room conjuring up her worst fears. After the allotted time, she could go about her day. I also asked her to keep track of her fears in a small notebook, which we would later discuss in therapy. I saw Jeanette every two weeks, and by writing down her fears in her notebook and deliberately summoning them up in her room, she slowly managed to take control of her anxiety. Since her fears were what had been keeping her awake and steering her toward playing Internet games until late at night, she was sleeping a little better now and looked more rested. Slowly, her grades began to improve. She had stopped taking the medications because she felt they weren't helping her.

Jeanette's problems were not ADHD or clinical depression, even though her symptoms undoubtedly would have fit the *DSM-5* criteria for both. Her problems were anxieties triggered by long-term tensions in her family. To escape, she started spending too much time gaming on the Internet. This resulted in sleep deprivation, which is often mistaken for ADHD in teenagers. And her insomnia led to a vicious cycle of Internet addiction. Gaming at night can even exacerbate depression in teens. According to a recent study at Johns Hopkins University, exposure to light at night from electronic screens can elevate levels of a stress hormone and lead to depression and learning problems. A psychiatrist could not get to the source of Jeanette's problems by going through a checklist of symptoms for ADHD or depression.

The best solution for Jeanette was not an endless series of medications, which ultimately failed to help her. What actually worked was giving her the tools she needed to help her with her anxieties and helping her parents to address their own problems outside of Jeanette's hearing. These interventions helped her focus on her school-work better than pharmaceutical drugs.

As much as teens are glued to their games and their smartphones, gaming is not always the cause of their problems. Instead, it may be a way to retreat from painful problems in their family or with friends. Excessive gaming can also be the result of loneliness, the feeling of not fitting in with any particular group in middle school or high school. In Jeanette's case, she had pulled away from most of her friends because their constant conversations about college made her feel like an outsider. She knew she would be going to the local community college, and she was afraid that the kids she had known all her life looked down on her because of this. It was easier to hide out in the virtual world in her room.

Therapy with Jeanette, which took a little more than a year, was a combination of shoring up her self-confidence and constantly reassuring her that she could have a bright future despite her day-to-day misery. Trust was a big hurdle at first because she was so afraid of people judging her. I often drew her out about video games. Letting her explain her favorite games to me made her feel that she was an expert and had something to offer me. She enjoyed these conversations and over time she came to trust me. Although she rarely smiled, I could sometimes make her laugh by tapping into her sarcastic sense of humor. Jeanette graduated with her class and now goes to a local community college, where she has made a few new friends. She is looking forward to transferring to a four-year school and plans to major in journalism. Occasionally she comes to see me for "tune-up" sessions, but in general she is doing well.

Media Violence

Along with video and computer game addiction, media violence is a major parental concern. Whether or not there is a connection between violent games and violent behavior is an ongoing controversy among researchers and politicians. In 2011, through the efforts of thousands of concerned parents in California, the state passed a law that limited purchases of violent games to persons eighteen and older. But the law was famously slapped down by the United States Supreme Court. In *Brown v. Entertainment Merchants Association*, the Court ruled by a 7 to 2 majority that violent games were subject to First Amendment protection. Writing for the majority opinion, Justice Antonin Scalia noted that depictions of violence have never been subject to government regulation. Scalia observed that the classic stories from *Grimm's Fairy Tales* like "Snow White," "Cinderella," and "Hansel and Gretel" are violent and gory.

But what Justice Scalia failed to observe is that these stories are qualitatively different from the fast-paced interactive video games that engage children in killing, maiming, and ravaging as entertainment. In the *Grimm's* tales, innocent children inevitably win out over evil villains, not through violence but through their own cleverness and with the help of forces for good. Hansel and Gretel outwit the wicked witch by leaving a trail of bread crumbs through the forest so they can find their way home. Snow White escapes her evil stepmother's plan to murder her with the help of magical childlike creatures, the seven dwarfs. These stories do not entice children to engage in murderous, brutal, or vengeful acts. On the contrary, children usually identify with the good characters, who are often innocent but clever children or small animals like fish and frogs with magical powers.

As for the Supreme Court decision, Justice Stephen Breyer wrote a dissenting minority opinion, pointing out that the Court's majority decision conflicted with its previous rulings regulating sales to children of publications containing nudity. "What sense does it make," Justice Breyer asked, "to forbid selling to a thirteen-year-old boy a magazine with an image of a nude woman, while protecting a sale to that thirteen-year-old of an interactive video game in which he actively, but virtually, binds and gags the woman, then tortures and kills her?"

Justice Clarence Thomas also wrote a separate dissenting opinion that upheld the sovereign right of parents to protect their children from "speech" that might do them harm. Thomas cited the Founding Fathers' belief that parents should have complete authority over their minor children and have the responsibility to direct their children's development. In his interpretation, the intent of the First Amendment "does not include a right to speak to minors (or a right of minors to access speech) without going through the minors' parents or guardians." In a similar vein, the Parents Television Council called the Supreme Court decision a "constitutionally protected end-run on parental authority." Leland Yee, the California state senator who wrote the law, declared that the ruling in the *Brown* case was just one more instance of the Supreme Court putting the interests of corporate America before the well-being of children.

The Supreme Court decision placed the full burden of responsibility on parents for monitoring the quality of the video games their children play. It's true that parents are the best observers of their own kids. Just as my husband and I noticed a change in our sons' moods after they spent long stretches of time on a (non-graphic) video game, parents in California were noticing the effects of violent games on their kids' moods and behaviors. But parents have a tough time enforcing rules about video or computer games. They can protect their children in their own home, but kids can still play violent games at their friends' houses or on the sly without parental supervision.

As the Supreme Court indicated in its decision, research on the topic is not conclusive. Whether violent games cause violent acts is a subject of debate from the halls of academia to the corridors of government. In 2013, President Obama ordered the Centers for Disease Control and Prevention to investigate the relationship between video games and real-world violence. Senator Jay Rockefeller introduced a bill the same year calling for the National Academy of Sciences to research the effects of violent video games on young children. The Senate has not yet acted on this bill. In response to these actions, the Entertainment Software Association issued a statement that scientific research has "proven" that entertainment does not cause real-world violent behavior.

But the case is far from closed. A new study in Singapore, published in *JAMA Pediatrics* in March 2014, suggests that children who play violent video games may have an increased rate of aggressive thoughts, which can lead to more aggressive behavior. In the study of three thousand children ages eight to seventeen, researchers found that children who spent more time playing violent video games exhibited increased signs of violent behavior, such as hitting, shoving, and pushing, three years after the study began. Children who played more violent video games tended to have more fantasies about violence and to believe that violence in real life was more acceptable. Researchers concluded that the children's aggressive behaviors stemmed from this increase in aggressive thoughts. For example, they were more likely to regard someone bumping into them as a hostile act. One researcher said this may be because the gaming led them to view violent solutions as more reasonable. On the other hand, children who decreased video game time showed less aggressive behavior.

The Singapore study of course has its critics, and the debate goes on. Research studies are criticized or defended, depending on one's personal motivations, values, and financial interests. In the end, parents are left to make their own decisions about their kids' exposure to violent video and computer games. Without protective regulation by government agencies, game corporations are left to pursue profits without regard for the well-being of society. While the jury is still out on the effect of video games on real-world violence, common sense suggests that parents would do well to err on the side of caution. They should limit their children's exposure to violent video games just as they would limit their exposure to violent movies and television shows and their younger children's exposure to fast-paced cartoons.

The view that ADHD-type behavior is a real disease entity and not merely on a continuum with normal childhood behavior encourages the use of drug treatment. But we know that drug treatment is not always the first choice of many parents or even doctors these days, as they become informed about the misinformation and unreliable research about ADHD. In the next chapter, I discuss parenting and family interventions that I have found effective in helping children with inattentiveness and/or hyperactive behavior.

NINE

Time-Tested Tactics for Good Parenting

The child supplies the power but the
parents have to do the steering.

• BENJAMIN SPOCK

Sitting in a room with Ricky was like watching a beam of light bounc-ing from every surface. A lanky boy with blond hair and blue eyes, Ricky was in constant motion, darting from one side of my office to the other and talking nonstop. He asked permission to use my computer and, after I let him, he brought up a recent music video he had up-loaded to his YouTube music channel. He was playing the trumpet with a swirl of changing colors in the background. The video was an impres-sive piece of work for a twenty-year-old, let alone a ten-year-old.

Ricky's parents had brought him to therapy because his high energy and impulsiveness had been disrupting his classroom. He got good grades but lately had been blurting out answers before his teacher called on him. He couldn't restrain himself from chatting with his class-mates. He hummed to himself and sometimes drummed on his desk, seemingly oblivious to the fact that he was distracting other pupils. Ricky was so excited about making music videos that he sometimes forgot to do his homework.

Ricky's teacher liked him and recognized his extraordinary talent. She had found ways to let him move around during the school day, such as appointing him attendance monitor. Every morning he took the attendance sheets from the classroom to the principal's office. His teacher had also put him in charge of bringing in and putting away the equipment after physical education class. But she worried about how he would do the following year when he entered middle school. She doubted middle school teachers would be as accommodating as she had been with Ricky's classroom behavior and missing homework assignments.

Ricky Finds His Own Solution

"Do you ever calm down and relax?" I asked Ricky in our first session. "When I'm asleep," he said, grinning. "Only when you're asleep?" I asked with a laugh. He pondered this for a moment and then his freckled face broke into a wily smile. "Also when I'm in science class because I'm asleep then, too," he answered. Ricky is a born charmer. He's one of the most endearing children I've ever met, although to his parents he must be exhausting. "I've found another way to relax," he told me. "What's that?" I asked. "I found a video on YouTube that plays the sound of waves. When I close my eyes and listen to the waves, I feel calm." Better than Ritalin, I say to myself. Ricky seems to have found a form of meditation for himself. "Do you want to hear it?" he asked. "Sure," I said. He found the video and we sat quietly listening to the waves. Ricky stopped talking. His eyes were closed. His feet stopped tapping. He was still.

I suspected that underneath his charm and brilliance, Ricky was feeling anxiety and emotional pain. Once we developed a rapport, I asked him if he was worried about either of his parents. I ask my young patients this question because sometimes children, especially if they are bright and sensitive, pick up on a parent's anxiety or depression. These children then behave in ways that "help" a parent by deflecting the parent's attention away from the more serious problem. "Mommy is unhappy at work," Ricky told me. "She doesn't like her job anymore. Sometimes she cries. And she yells at me for playing video games too much." "I'm sure she yells because she is stressed out," I reassured him. "Maybe I can help her deal with the stress." "Yeah," Ricky said.

I asked Ricky to sit in my waiting room while I talked with his parents, Kevin and Edie. They filled me in on the story. Four years earlier, when Ricky was six, his teacher, school counselor, and principal tried to convince Edie and Kevin that Ricky had ADHD. Even his grandmother, who is a special education teacher, thought he needed medication. They took him to the pediatrician and, after reading a report from Ricky's teacher, the doctor wrote a prescription for Adderall. Kevin and Edie didn't fill the prescription. They were too worried about the side effects, which they'd seen described in great detail on the Internet. Instead, they took Ricky to an educational therapist for a psycho-educational assessment. The two-day testing showed that Ricky's IQ topped 150— putting him in the top 1 percent of the population. He was exceptionally gifted and his parents thought he might be bored by the work in his first-grade classroom. Research shows that behaviors associated with giftedness—like poor attention and low tolerance for tasks that seem to the child to be boring or irrelevant—are associated with diagnoses of ADHD.

Kevin and Edie set about finding activities that would challenge Ricky. They enrolled him in soccer as an outlet for his energy. They bought a secondhand piano and found a piano teacher for him. They took him to the library on Saturdays and helped him choose books that interested him. The educational therapist had recommended that Ricky's parents keep the atmosphere at home as calm as possible. They took her advice and became more consistent about enforcing rules about video games and television. When parents are consistent about rules, their anger at the child's behavior doesn't heat up to the boiling point and they are less likely to explode. Ricky was still high energy and nervous, but with consistently enforced rules his behavior calmed down quite a bit. Then, about a year before I met the family, he started blurting out answers in class and not finishing his assignments. What had happened in the family around this time? I wondered.

I asked them about their work. Kevin taught music at the neighborhood high school and gave cello lessons to a few students in the evenings. Edie was a social worker for twenty-five hours a week at a local hospital. Kevin drove Ricky to school every morning and Edie picked him up and took him to soccer practice and music lessons. I could see that they were devoted parents. Kevin had an older son in college from a previous marriage. "Ricky loves him," Edie told me. I asked Edie if she likes her job. "I used to love my job," she said. "But a year ago I got a new boss. She's really hard to work for." Edie's voice started to tremble and her eyes filled with tears. "Sometimes I wish I didn't have to work, but we need the money. It's so frustrating because I used to love my job and the people I worked with." Kevin cut her off. "I think she should quit," he said. "Her boss is way too difficult and demanding. This year has been a nightmare. We can manage without Edie working until she finds another job. Meanwhile, I can take on a few more cello students."

"Do you think my being unhappy at work is affecting Ricky?" Edie asked me. I explained that children are finely attuned to their parents' troubles. Ricky might have been feeling anxious about his mother's situation. In a loving home, I explained to them, children want to protect their parents just as much as the parents want to protect their children. Children often pick up on a parent's anxiety or depression and sometimes act out to distract them from their worries.

Staying Positive

"I'm going to give you a simple strategy," I said to Edie. "I'd like to ask you not to say anything negative about your work or your boss in Ricky's hearing. If you could say just one good thing about your day it would help a lot. And of course it has to be at least partially true. You could say that you went out to lunch with a coworker or that your boss was nicer to you. You could say that you enjoyed a few minutes of gardening before work. But you have to say one positive thing about your day and nothing negative." I added, "Ricky is really bright, so don't be too obvious about it."

"If it will help Ricky, I'll do it," Edie said. I am pretty sure it will help. This strategy is simple but powerful. Of course, the *"I had a good day"* strategy was a short-term solution for this family. The longer-term answer was for Edie to resolve her job situation so she could be happier. I also suggested that Edie and Kevin be careful about yelling at Ricky. Edie admitted she had been having a hard time enforcing rules about video games. Sometimes she lost patience and yelled. We decided on a plan. Ricky would be allowed a half hour after school to work on his music videos or do whatever he wanted before starting his homework. After he finished his homework, he would be allowed one more hour of gaming or videos. "We can also start reading books together again," Kevin said. "That's a good idea," I said. Reading alone or with a parent can be much more calming than watching fast-paced screens. I asked their permission to conduct gentle hypnosis or mindfulness training with Ricky, to support his efforts to calm himself. They were more than happy with this idea.

In the next two sessions, I met with Ricky by himself. I used a mild form of guided imagery to put him in a light trance. Ricky closed his eyes and soon his body became perfectly still. The only movement was his soft breathing. When I brought him out of the trance, he said he felt calmer. He told me he would like to go back to that peaceful place at home by himself. In the second session, we began with guided imagery for a few minutes. Ricky was able to sit in a chair for the rest of the session and didn't dart around the room. When I saw Edie and Kevin a month later, they told me they were seeing a difference. Ricky was calmer and less impulsive. His teacher had said he was getting better about not blurting out answers and not distracting his classmates. This encouraged Edie to continue saying positive things about her day to Ricky. She had also updated her résumé and was starting to look for a different job.

I met with Ricky and his parents over the course of six months, alternating between individual sessions with Ricky and meetings with his parents. One day Ricky confided that he wished his father would take him fishing during the summer. I thought this was a good idea because I know that being out in nature has a soothing effect on children. Kevin was more than happy to take Ricky fishing. That summer, they enjoyed two overnight camping trips on the shore of a lake and they fished every day. By the time he started middle school, Ricky was doing much better. His school offers honors classes in math and English for gifted students, and Ricky easily made the cut. He is also taking a seventh-grade computer class. Ricky is still an active and energetic boy but he is able to control his impulsivity in the classroom.

The Emperor's New Clothes

ADHD is the embodiment of the story "The Emperor's New Clothes." People with money and power can create realities and make the public believe that these "realities" exist independently. We start to see the world the way those in power want us to see it. But it doesn't have to be this way. If we realize that children can be overactive and impulsive for any number of reasons, we can avoid reducing their behavior to a simplistic diagnosis of ADHD. As I've observed, behaviors like Ricky's, which others may interpret as a medical condition, can be turned around by making changes in the child's home life and by making accommodations at school.

This chapter offers parents a different lens through which they can view their children's difficult behaviors. I offer strategies that are deceptively simple but remarkably effective in changing behaviors that doctors define as ADHD. These strategies put the authority of children's emotional and behavioral well-being back where it has traditionally belonged: into the hands of parents.

The strategies in this chapter will not turn your home into Camelot overnight, but I promise that if you make them part of your daily routine you will see a remarkable difference in your child in as little as a few weeks. Even if your son or daughter is taking medication for ADHD, these tools will help. If you are considering medication, try these tools before taking that step. I suggest that you don't start with all of the strategies at once. Begin with one and add a new one every few days. Be patient. The strategies take a little time to work, and they are different from the typical techniques outlined in parenting books. They are based on family-systems therapy and leverage the natural strength of the family to help a child. Until we know for certain the long-term effects of ADHD drugs on developing brains, we must take a cautious stance on their use and try other interventions instead.

STRATEGY 1: "I HAD A GOOD DAY"

This is the first strategy I prescribed to Edie. The idea is that parents say only positive things about their lives in front of their child. If you've been passed over for that promised promotion or your new boss is a tyrant, keep these issues away from the dinner table. Every day, make a point of saying one good thing about your day in front of your child. This means parents have to highlight simple things in their life that make them feel good, even if they have to use a magnifying glass to find them. You'd be surprised at how many young children tell me that "Daddy takes six pills every day for his heart" or "Mommy has a mean boss." I'm not saying you should lie to your child or create false rainbows, but be aware that your mood affects your kids. An added bonus of this strategy is that by focusing on the good things in your life, you wind up feeling happier.

That said, more than one parent I've seen in therapy has objected to this strategy. They believe parents should not protect kids from the harsh realities of life. My answer is that *if* a child is having problems, then the child should be protected from parental worries as much as possible. If a child is *not* having problems, then parents can share a small amount of negative information if they want to. If a child is having problems, she should not hear anything negative about a parent's health. Instead, she should hear: "I had my checkup today and the doctor said I was in perfect health," or "I haven't had any pain in my back for three months. I feel great since I've been going to yoga," or "I feel so much better since I've been working out at the gym."

I'm reminded of a seven-year-old girl named Lori whose personality changed overnight. She started having tantrums and refused to do what her parents asked her. Even the simplest requests caused a meltdown. A once sweet, cooperative child had changed into a monster. When I asked Lori what was worrying her, she told me that her mother had recently had stomach surgery. The idea of a doctor cutting her mother open with a knife was terrifying to Lori and caused her severe anxiety.

Of course, how much information you share with your child depends on the child's age. It's fine to tell a young child that Mommy is in the hospital for a few days, but it is not necessary to describe the details of a procedure that might frighten the child. One mother who had surgery for breast cancer told her ten-year-old daughter that the doctor took a piece of tissue from her chest. She did not mention cancer at all. She assured her daughter that the surgery was successful and that she would be fine. A parent might choose to share more details about a surgery with a teenager, though even then she should temper her explanation with words of reassurance.

Parents should not share their own troubles with the child as they would with a friend. Your child is not your confidant. If Dad is battling with his boss, he should take a few minutes to calm down before walking into the house. One father sat in his car and listened to music for ten minutes before pulling into his driveway in the evening. Another father decided to go to the gym after work for a brief workout to decompress from the stress of the day. Child psychiatrist Bruce Perry, who does not believe that ADHD is a real illness, observes that if a parent is feeling anxiety, a child may pick up the feeling and start to feel anxious as well. That is exactly what I see in the families I treat. Bad feelings are contagious, but so are positive ones. Of course, sometimes having to explain to a child that a grandmother is ill or that a grandfather is in the hospital is necessary, especially if parents must travel out of town to visit their mother or father. Again, the amount of detail that parents share depends on the age of the child.

STRATEGY 2: MAKE MINDFULNESS OR MEDITATION PART OF YOUR LIFE

One of the best things parents can do for their children is to take care of their own mental health. I often recommend yoga or meditation to parents who are feeling overwhelmed. These practices, also called "mindfulness," teach you to quiet your mind by focusing on your breathing. The term "mindfulness" comes from the Buddhist tradition and a translation of the Sanskrit word *smrti*, which means "a heightened attentiveness to the present moment." I discovered the practice of mindfulness when my children were young and I felt stressed out most of the time. When I found myself yelling at my kids, I went to a therapist who suggested I practice mindfulness. I read everything I could find on Buddhist meditation and listened to a tape the therapist had suggested. It took some practice, but I found that when I was able to focus my attention on my breathing and banish the stray thoughts and feel-ings that popped into my awareness, I felt calmer and more relaxed.

Mindfulness, as ten-year-old Ricky discovered for himself, can also help overly active children slow down and control their impulsiveness. Some doctors think mindfulness may be an alternative to ADHD medi-cations. A large study, published in 2013 in the *Journal of the American Academy of Child and Adolescent Psychiatry*, by University of California professor James Swanson and his team, found that ADHD medications may help children in the short term but that the effectiveness of the drugs usually wanes by the third year. He suggests that mindfulness might help ADHD children more effectively than drugs in the long term because this practice helps children learn to manage their own behavior and focus their attention.

STRATEGY 3: DON'T ARGUE IN FRONT OF THE KIDS

The third strategy is simple: If parents need to quarrel, they should do so out of earshot of the kids. A long history of research has found that parental conflict has a negative impact on children's psychological de-velopment. And in my own clinical experience I have found that hear-ing parents fight is the number one cause of aggressive and violent behavior in children, as well as the source of many attention and focus-ing problems. In children's vivid imaginations, parental disagreements may seem more significant than they really are. Children worry that re-peated bickering may signal that divorce is imminent. Today, most chil-dren have friends whose parents are divorced and can't help but worry that their parents might also split up. The no-arguing-in-front-of-the-kids rule is especially important if parents are separated or divorced.

Renegotiating a healthy co-parenting relationship after a divorce is one of the most important (yet difficult) things you can do for your child. You don't have to be friends with your ex, but it's best to have a civilized relationship at least with respect to your child so that the child is not burdened by your ongoing anger.

All couples argue, especially with the stress that so many parents experience these days. An argument may not mean the end of the world to you, but it might well be disturbing to your child. It's also best not to contradict the other parent in front of the kids. Wait until you have a chance to talk privately and then express your disagreements to each other. Of course, this is an ideal scenario for parents and not always possible in the heat of anger. But it's a good rule to keep in mind.

The bickering-parent problem is compounded when parents disagree about rules concerning their child. A child can easily step in and take over power in the family by forming an alliance with the more lenient parent. When parents are not united, the power vacuum is all too readily filled by an *enfant roi*. This brings us to the next strategy about maintaining a healthy balance of family relationships

STRATEGY 4: KEEP THE FAMILY HIERARCHY

In family-systems theory we talk about the *family hierarchy* and *boundaries*. A natural family hierarchy is one in which parents are in charge of the children and not the other way around. This also means that parents must keep their relationship strong and healthy by occasionally spending time together without the children. Some parents look at me in surprise when I recommend they go out on dates alone together. "But we go out as a *family*," they tell me. That's not the same thing.

Spending quality time together as a family is important and (let's hope) enjoyable, but it's just as important for parents to nurture their own relationship by having quality time together without the kids. This time away charges parents' batteries so that when they return they can present a united front to their children. Kids who are jumpy or irritable are more likely to settle down when their parents are on the same page.

Many parents extend the concept of date nights to taking weekends or short vacations without the children. These little getaways are nothing short of miraculous in improving and sustaining a family's mental health. I'm not saying parents should hop on the next plane to Hawaii. I am just emphasizing the importance of parents carving out enjoyable time for themselves as a couple, leaving their children with grandparents or a trusted babysitter. The getaway doesn't have to be expensive. It can be as simple as a camping trip.

There's no doubt that babies and toddlers put a strain on a relationship. The French even have a phrase for this—the "baby-clash," which refers to the risk of parents separating in the first few years after their baby is born. I have seen some young couples go into a state of near shock during the early stages of parenthood. A "fight or flight" reaction sets in as they struggle to make joint decisions about child care, sleeping arrangements, discipline, changing diapers, and even the role of grandparents. One young mother never recovered from the strain of having both her mother and mother-in-law in her house when her son was born. For the next two years she blamed her husband for the stress his mother had caused her. Even after a year of counseling, the couple divorced shortly before their son's third birthday. They were casualties of the baby-clash. It's best when couples see the baby-clash coming and discuss potential sources of stress in advance.

STRATEGY 5: CHILDREN NEED STRUCTURE

Most parenting experts agree that children do better when their life is predictable and their day has limits and structure. Some examples of structure are pre-established mealtimes, bedtime, the time to get up in the morning, and the time at which homework must be started. Some families find that having a weekly cleanup during which children spend an hour straightening up their room provides a good structure. The structure of family mealtimes is important for children. This is a time for them to learn good table manners (which includes not texting their friends from the dinner table) and healthy eating habits. Serve the same food for everyone and insist that your child at least taste everything at the table. Your son might not like asparagus quiche or arugula salad the first time he tries them, but in time his taste might change. My kids used to wince at the sight of a mushroom, but today they enjoy portobello omelets.

Within the boundaries of a structured day, a child should have plenty of choices. For example, your daughter may be expected to clean her room on Saturdays, but she can decide what time to clean it. Your son may not be allowed to eat cookies or other sweets whenever he wants to at any time of day, but he may have a sweet at snack time or for dessert after dinner. Bedtime may be eight o'clock, but on weekends or when the child attends an evening birthday party, you can agree on a later time. When parents provide limits and don't give in to whining and screaming, children learn patience. They learn to tolerate a little bit of frustration, which is an important skill in life. Living with structure from an early age, children find comfort in rules, and parents naturally maintain and evolve these rules as the child develops.

STRATEGY 6: DISCIPLINE MEANS EDUCATION

Much of what is labeled ADHD can be corrected when parents put a good system of discipline in place. I don't really like the word "discipline," which connotes "punishment." I prefer the word the French use, *education*, which has the same meaning as discipline. "Discipline" is derived from the Latin word *disciplina*, which means "instruction" or "education." When parents put rules and limits into place, they are educating a child on good behavior and good manners.

Whatever rules you decide on, the most important thing is to enforce them calmly, consistently, and immediately. That means no yelling, no spanking, and no idle threats. Yelling and spanking make a child feel anxious and seldom do any good. Idle threats make a child laugh. "You're grounded for a year" will never work because your child knows you won't follow through on this threat. A time-out for a toddler or telling an older child that she is grounded from an important birthday party are more realistic and enforceable consequences.

Both parents need to be on the same page about discipline and to back each other up. This is often more easily said than done. It means, for one thing, that they must discuss the rules in private and come to an agreement on how they will "educate" their child in good behavior. I've seen situations in which a child is acting so out of control that the parents think he might be too "mentally ill" to learn good behavior. Because the child has a "mental disorder," they believe he should not be held accountable and that only medicine will help him control himself. These parents back off enforcing rules because they think disciplining their child means punishing her for behavior over which she has no control.

But loving a child does not mean you let him run wild until he becomes diagnosable. I will always remember the words of my children's preschool teacher, who was an exceptionally warm and caring person. "Love means discipline," she told me. Love means not only making your child happy, but also taking the time and trouble to educate the child in appropriate behavior. I have seen the terrible consequences when one parent is too softhearted to discipline and the other parent cringes at seeing the child grow up without limits but cannot do anything about it. In this kind of situation a child truly becomes an *enfant roi*, running the show because she has successfully split the authority of her parents.

Here are six tried and tested techniques for "educating" a child in good behavior.

First, create clear rules and explain them to your child. You might even want to post them on the child's bedroom door or on the refrigerator. A good example is the issue of respect, a topic that often comes up in therapy. Tell your child exactly what you mean by respect. For example: Respect means doing what parents ask you to do without arguing, name-calling, or using bad words. Then reward your child with reciprocal respect and praise when you catch him being respectful.

Kids are literal-minded so rules should be specific. Instead of saying that a child is responsible for cleaning her room, define exactly what you mean by "clean"—for example, bed made, no dirty clothes or towels on the floor, and belongings neatly put away in drawers or closets. For older children, "clean" can include vacuuming and dusting their room.

Second, use the count of three when your child disobeys, whines, argues, or has a meltdown. In our home, my husband came up with the "count of three" method, which worked very well with our children. If they did not do what we asked them to do by the time we counted to three, they got an immediate consequence. Fifteen years later, when parents asked me to recommend a good book on discipline, I discovered the book *1-2-3 Magic*, by Dr. Thomas Phelan, which describes a similar technique. By telling a child that you will discipline them after you count to three, you give him a couple of chances to contemplate the imminent consequence and shape up. If you get to three, you give a young child a time-out in her room or in a corner. For older children, you can take away video game privileges, confiscate their cell phone (or turn off their Internet service), or ground the child for a weekend. You do this while showing as little emotion as possible even though you are probably boiling inside.

For so-called ADHD kids, Phelan says, parents might have a hard time getting them to stay in their room for a time-out. He has a few gentle, though effective, solutions for this kind of situation. For young kids, he suggests standing in front of the door and holding it shut or blocking the child's exit with a gate that squeezes against the doorjambs. This solution is useful as long as the child is not able to climb over or knock down the gate. Another option is to start the time-out over if the child comes out of his room before the specified time. For kids who keep coming out or for older kids, Phelan even recommends locking their door.

Once children learn they must stay in their room, the tantrums will cease and they will accept the time-out. Phelan argues that although locking a child in his room seems harsh, it does not harm a child as much as endless yelling, arguing, and shouting matches. He points out that many children will test the counting to see if parents really mean it.

If parents follow through consistently, children will eventually stop test-ing. I have recommended *1-2-3 Magic* to hundreds of parents over the years and have found that when it's used consistently and calmly, the counting technique actually does work like magic.

Third, make a star chart or use a point system. Star charts are useful for reinforcing children's positive behaviors, such as being ready for school on time, brushing their teeth, or having a day without incidents at school. You put a calendar on the refrigerator door or in the child's room where it is in plain view. Every day that the child completes the desired behavior, he gets a gold star. If he gets four out of five stars on weekdays, then on weekends he gets rewarded with a treat. The treat can be a special excursion to the ice cream shop, a small toy, having a friend over for pizza, or even being allowed to stay up past bedtime. It's good to keep the chart simple and start out by targeting the one behavior that is most important to you and easy for the child to learn. For many parents, that means being ready to go to school on time. For other parents, it's having the child get through the school day without any reports of misbehavior.

For older children and more serious problem behaviors, a "token economy," also known as a "point system," can replace the star chart. A child can gain points for positive behaviors like cleaning her room, get-ting her homework done without prompting, or getting ready for school on time. When a child does not do what is expected of her, she loses points. To earn privileges, the child must accumulate a specified number of points. For especially obnoxious behavior, the child's school may go to a point system as well. If a child does not behave well enough at school to earn the specified number of points, she loses privileges like recess or field trips.

With star charts and points, as with counting, the most important thing is for parents to follow through consistently as a united front. One mother was reluctant to deprive her sixth grader of a family trip to visit his grandparents in Paris. However, when her son did not earn enough points, she canceled the trip for the whole family. Her son eventually stopped his obnoxious behavior when he finally understood that his parents meant what they said, even if the whole family had to suffer the consequences. The family then rescheduled the trip for the following summer.

Fourth, devise effective consequences. Many parenting experts urge parents to use *natural consequences* to teach children about the effects of their decisions in the real world. For example, if your seventh grader is supposed to make her school lunches, the natural consequence for forgetting to pack her lunch is that she will be hungry at lunchtime. To some parents, the thought of their little dear missing a meal is unbearable. Recently, however, American parents have come under criticism for overcoddling and overprotecting children. (As a parent, I am not exempt from this failing.) Parental overprotectiveness is well intentioned but it can lead to a young adult who is unable to cope with life's hardships. Instead of worrying that a seventh grader will be hungry at lunchtime while other kids are eating, a parent who trusts her kid's resourcefulness (maybe a friend will share some of her lunch or a teacher will lend her lunch money) sends the message to the child that her parents believe in her ability to think for herself and find solutions to problems.

Along with time-outs and removing privileges like screen time and sleepovers, giving a child what I call a "helping chore" is a surprisingly effective consequence for misbehavior. A helping chore is an age-appropriate task that helps parents—for a young child, picking up toys, wiping the kitchen table or refrigerator with a sponge, dusting, or setting the table. The chore should take five to ten minutes and be supervised by a parent. An older child can rake leaves, help wash the car, or empty the dishwasher. For an older child, the chore should take fifteen to twenty minutes. Often a child will gain more from doing a "helping chore" than by losing a privilege.

Fifth, don't lecture your child. Be short and to the point when you are "educating" him. Say no when you have to, but say it quickly and with conviction. Remember, you are not giving a lecture or opening a negotiation. Explain the reason for the no if your child asks, but if she keeps asking you why, then say, "We'll talk about that later," and be prepared with your answer. Children do best when parents are decisive. As Pamela Druckerman observes in *Bringing Up Bébé*, parents must be confident in their decisions and give a non-ambivalent delivery. Look your child in the eye, kneeling down to his level if you have to, and explain the rule. Remember, your child needs to recognize that you are in charge. Children feel more secure when they know you are steering the ship on a clear course with a firm hand. Of course, you want to say yes to your child as often as possible when the request is reasonable.

Sixth, an ounce of prevention is worth forty milligrams of Adderall. The earlier parents begin to educate a child in good behavior, the less likely the child will rebel or need medication to control himself later on. Around the age of the "terrible twos" (though it can be earlier or later), a child will begin to test parental limits. He needs to learn for himself what these limits really mean and if he can bend them to his own will. If parents don't set limits when a child is young, they will have a tough time imposing them later on. Ten-year-old Tommy, a patient of mine who was the very picture of a child king, was born when his mother was forty-two after she had undergone infertility treatments for several years. She loved him so much that she didn't like to discipline him, despite her husband's protests that boys need discipline.

When he was seven, Tommy's pediatrician diagnosed him with ADHD and prescribed Adderall. By age nine, Tommy was so defiant and argumentative at home and at school that his parents took him to a child psychiatrist. The psychiatrist diagnosed Tommy with oppositional defiant disorder (ODD) as well as ADHD. He raised the dosage of Adderall and also prescribed Zoloft, an antidepressant, and Intuniv, a blood pressure medication that is sometimes used to treat ADHD-type symptoms. The psychiatrist also thought Tommy needed more discipline at home and recommended several parenting books. When Tommy's parents started to set limits and follow through with consequences, Tommy became so angry that one day after his mother took away his cell phone, he bit her arm so badly that she needed stitches.

If Tommy's parents had committed to educating him in good behavior earlier, they wouldn't have had to make the sudden drastic changes that precipitated this extreme incident. Certainly, as a child progresses through different stages of development some unruly behaviors may emerge. The question for parents is: Have they prepared for these eventualities with a clear plan for discipline? Or have they, like so many American parents, allowed their children unrestrained gratification of their desires?

Along with using these strategies, parents can head off an ADHD diagnosis by making sure that their child has plenty of sleep, a good breakfast of natural unprocessed foods high in protein and low in sugar, ample opportunities for physical exercise and outdoor play, limited time on electronic screens, and appropriate doses of praise. If parents need additional support, they can enroll in a parent-training program like the Incredible Years or the many other parenting programs that are springing up in the United States. Children, especially preschoolers, also need plenty of time for unstructured play. Children begin fidgeting when they do not have enough time to move around during their day. Instead of rushing a child into school right after his fifth birthday, consider giving him the gift of extra time.

Exercise as Medication for ADHD

Along with parent-training programs, researchers in the United States and abroad are looking at a variety of other interventions as an alternative to medication for kids with ADHD-type symptoms. A 2012 Danish study found that simply walking to school can help a child with attention problems. Professor Niels Egelund, of Aarhus University, observed, "The exercise you get from transporting yourself to school reflects on your ability to concentrate for about four hours into the school day."

A British study came to similar conclusions. Dr. William Bird, a physician and the founder of the company that conducted the study, suggested three reasons why walking to school may have this effect. First, physical activity improves brain elasticity, which allows children to learn more easily. Second, contact with the natural environment has a proven calming effect on children. And third, exercise releases endorphins (neurotransmitters that produce a feeling of well-being), which makes children feel more relaxed. Children also reported another benefit. Walking to school gave them a chance to spend more time with their friends and to make new friends.

A 2013 study by researchers at the University of Illinois found that after twenty minutes of brisk walking or jogging on treadmills, children who had been diagnosed with ADHD, as well as a group of "normal" children, significantly increased their scores on a complicated test. John Ratey, an associate professor of psychiatry at Harvard, suggests that parents think of exercise as medication for ADHD. Ratey believes that physical activity "improves mood and cognitive performance by triggering the brain to release dopamine and serotonin, similar to the way that stimulant medications like Adderall do."

In this pharmaceutical era, our image of childhood has dramatically changed. Doctors prescribe stimulants to mold children's behavior and enhance their cognitive performance from preschool to high school and beyond. As a society we have taken a wrong turn and are badly in need of a new paradigm for child mental health. In the next chapter, I will show how family therapy and cross-cultural wisdom can lead us in a new direction.

TEN Protecting Children in the Age of Adderall

> I want to thank my mom and dad up in
> heaven for disobeying the doctor's or-
> ders and not medicating their hyperac-
> tive daughter and finding out what
> she's into instead.
>
> • AUDRA MCDONALD

Every new generation of parents faces its unique challenges. But one dilemma that confronts parents in every epoch is how (and how much) to protect our children. Parents have a natural instinct to keep their children safe and protect them as much as possible from life's hardships. Yet, many experts argue that today's parents have gone overboard and are not allowing their children to take enough risks or face enough obstacles on their own. A bevy of recent parenting books addressed to overly protective parents are raising the battle cry of "retreat." Teach your kids to look both ways before they cross the street, but don't try to smooth over all of life's rough patches for them. Helicopter parenting only makes kids feel helpless and powerless. Even worse, it deprives them of the emotional resources they need to become self-sufficient adults. Kids need to handle a few bumps in the road by themselves in order to learn resilience and self-reliance.

In today's world, though, a new threat looms that was unknown to previous generations of parents. Keeping kids safe today is not just about teaching them not to talk to strangers, walking them to school, or keeping an eye on them from the kitchen window while they play outside. It's not just about keeping kids away from the junk foods and junk media that are available to them everywhere they go. The real challenge for parents today is protecting kids from our culture's casual acceptance of behavior-modifying psychiatric drugs for children. These drugs not only carry significant health risks, but they also make a child feel like he has to depend on a drug to get through his day. This teaches a child the opposite of self-reliance.

Rachel

Eight-year-old Rachel, a patient of mine, was typical of a child diagnosed with ADHD. Rachel's parents, Jack and Eileen, first came to my office on a warm afternoon in early spring. Rachel was in school, and Eileen was planning to pick her up after our session. When I greeted the couple in the waiting room, Jack's eyes were glued to his smartphone. I put out my hand, and he quickly tucked the phone into his pocket, smiled, and shook my hand. Jack and Eileen were well-educated people and devoted parents. Jack was a software engineer and Eileen worked part-time from home as a graphic designer. Rachel was the oldest of their three children.

Jack spoke first, frequently touching the phone in his pocket as he talked. Ever since Rachel was in kindergarten, he explained, she had had behavior and attention issues. She also had angry episodes when she would throw things at her siblings or at children in her classroom. Now in second grade, she continued to wet the bed and had to wear diapers at night.

Eileen listened while Jack talked, but several times he cut her off when she tried to speak. Now she turned to me and continued the story. According to her teacher, Rachel was very bright, Eileen said, but her difficulty paying attention and focusing were preventing her from doing her best. Often she made careless mistakes on assignments even though she knew the answers. Capable of getting As, she was instead earning Bs and Cs, and even an occasional D.

Seeing their daughter struggle at school and worried about her escalating misbehavior, her parents decided to consult their pediatrician. After taking a history and talking with Rachel and her parents, the doctor diagnosed her with ADHD and prescribed Adderall XR. Eileen recognized the name "Adderall," since the children of two of her friends were taking it. She and Jack read about the many stimulant medications listed on the Internet, and they decided that the side effects of Adderall were acceptable if the drug helped Rachel do better at school.

From the day she began taking Adderall, Rachel started to focus better. She was more motivated in the classroom and seemed calmer at home. After about a week, however, Rachel started to have an adverse reaction to the drug. She had trouble falling asleep and said she felt like "bugs were crawling underneath her skin." Her parents called the pediatrician and he changed the prescription to Ritalin. Unfortunately, Ritalin had the same effect. It helped Rachel for a few days, and then made her feel agitated and "crazy." About one in a hundred children who take these drugs have side effects like these.

So the doctor tried Intuniv. Intuniv is not a stimulant and therefore he hoped it would have fewer side effects. Rachel tolerated this drug better, but there was no noticeable improvement in her behavior or attentiveness. Meanwhile, her angry outbursts had intensified to the point that one day she threw herself to the floor in a rage and clawed her mother when she tried to pick her up because she didn't want to go to gymnastics class.

Frightened by the intensity of Rachel's tantrums, Jack and Eileen made an appointment with a prominent child psychiatrist, well known as a specialist in ADHD. They traveled more than forty miles to see him. Half an hour later they came out of the doctor's office with a prescription for Risperdal, a powerful antipsychotic medication that is typically given to adults with serious mental illnesses, such as bipolar disorder or schizophrenia.

"Off Label" Antipsychotics

When Risperdal or other adult antipsychotics are prescribed "off label" to children with ADHD, it means that even though the FDA has not approved the drug for children who have an ADHD diagnosis, doctors are allowed to use their judgment to prescribe it anyway. Since the more typical ADHD medicines hadn't worked for Rachel, the new doctor decided to try a different class of drugs.

Eileen had never heard of Risperdal, so she set about researching it on the Internet. When she read that it was an antipsychotic drug with potential side effects of weight gain and increased risk of diabetes and cardiovascular problems, she was determined to keep her daughter off it. Eileen was already worried that Rachel was overweight for her age and height. She decided to get a second or even a third opinion before allowing her daughter to take Risperdal. Jack agreed. They looked into biofeedback, which carried a high price tag. Biofeedback is a technique that helps a person learn to control her body functions. Instruments measure physiological activity such as brain waves, heart function, breathing, muscle activity, and skin temperature. These instruments "feed back" information to the user. When Rachel's parents were told that biofeedback involved a family therapy component, they decided to try the family therapy first.

By the time I met them, Eileen and Jack had been through a lot and were growing more and more frustrated. Rachel was performing far below her ability at school, and her teacher was complaining about her out-of-control behavior. Jack and Eileen were open with me in the first session when I asked about their family life. As we talked, it became obvious that their marriage was unhappy and had been so for a long time. Jack told me in a voice filled with frustration that he was on the verge of asking for a divorce. Sure, Rachel's problems took a toll on him, but that wasn't the only reason for his unhappiness.

Jack and Eileen disagreed on just about every aspect of parenting: how much TV their children should be allowed to watch, the rules for bedtime and homework, what foods they should eat, and how to deal with Rachel's meltdowns. Eileen was more indulgent and allowed her daughter to have sugary desserts; Jack believed the sugar was contributing to Rachel's outbursts and inattentiveness. Eileen let Rachel watch commercial television programs for hours, while Jack thought she should, at most, be allowed to watch a program on PBS as a reward after finishing her homework. He preferred they watch no TV at all.

Disagreements about the children were not the only problem. Jack's restrictive vegan diet, which Eileen said he followed "obsessively," was driving her crazy because he made himself special meals and wouldn't eat with the children and her. "I don't want to watch them eating the garbage she gives them," Jack retorted. "Rachel is already overweight. And you can just watch her spiral out of control after she's had too much gluten and sugar."

Feeling as if I were stepping into a war zone, I gently explained to Eileen and Jack that we would have to resolve their disagreements about parenting in order for Rachel to start behaving better. Their first reaction, as is common for many parents, was incredulity. Since two medical doctors were working with the implicit notion that there was something biologically wrong with Rachel's brain chemistry, what on earth did their feuding or their different parenting styles have to do with their daughter's problems? I patiently explained that there was scant evidence for the brain-chemistry theory of ADHD. Medical researchers have not yet found a biochemical cause for ADHD on which they agree. Despite sixty years of heavily funded research, there is no laboratory test that indicates the presence or absence of ADHD in a child.

Giving Rachel a calm, structured home environment in which her parents agree on the rules of their household could help her more than any pill, I told her parents. Eileen had trouble accepting this. Jack, on the other hand, said that sometimes he thought Rachel didn't have ADHD at all. She can be such a sweet girl, he told me, and the next minute she seems to be "possessed by the devil." "You're not the first parent who has said that to me about their child," I assured Jack.

It was a challenge to help Jack and Eileen let go of the idea that their daughter's difficulties were caused by a defect in her brain, and I couldn't really blame them. That's the way our culture tends to view emotional problems these days. The brain has become the scapegoat for all sorts of childhood problems. So far, however, nobody had been able to explain to Rachel's parents exactly what the problem with their daughter's brain chemistry was. Although Jack and Eileen didn't quite believe what I was telling them, the other professionals had been of so little help that they were willing to hear me out.

I told them that the key to helping Rachel behave and feel better was for their relationship to improve and for them to become happier. Like most children of well-intentioned parents, Rachel desperately wanted her mother and father to be happy together. For years she had seen them at each other's throats and at times threatening divorce. Her parents' conflicts and unhappiness had created an atmosphere of chaos; they were the stressors that had put Rachel's behavior over the edge and made her have enough behavioral symptoms to be "diagnosable."

Jack and Eileen were giving each other grief, but it was their daughter who was feeling the most pain. Because Rachel could not find the words to voice the cause of her distress, it distracted her, irritated her, and manifested as inattentiveness and out-of-control behavior. For Rachel to get better, her parents' relationship had to be repaired. They had to come to an agreement on the rules of the household. They had to establish a stable family hierarchy. And they had to stop fighting with each other around Rachel. This was of course easier said than done.

Healing the Marriage

As we settled into the unique relationship that is family therapy, I realized that many years of buried resentments and anger would have to be aired. I met with Jack and Eileen alone for most of the sessions, bringing Rachel in only twice. Tough marital issues had to be resolved. Eileen and Jack still loved each other. Neither of them had cheated or betrayed the other's trust. The demands of their jobs and raising a family had pushed them apart and made them stop communicating in a healthy way. Their sex life had all but evaporated. While I struggled with the couple and made bits of progress, their fights abated and their household became less chaotic. Not surprisingly, Rachel slowly started to show improvement. Her angry episodes became rare, her grades improved, and she was calmer at school.

One afternoon about three months into our sessions, Rachel said with a smile: "Mommy and Daddy went out last night." She was feeling better because she could see that her parents were happier. The strident arguments had all but ceased. They were learning to compromise. Six months after her family first walked into my office, Rachel was behaving like a normal child. She is still strong-willed and likes to get what she wants. What child doesn't? On the spectrum of children, Rachel is relatively stubborn, relatively loud, and more than a little rambunctious. But she no longer has violent outbursts and has stopped wetting the bed. She is able to sit still in class and focus on her assignments, and she is getting As and Bs at school.

Most important, Rachel no longer qualifies for an ADHD diagnosis. Her symptoms were more a phase she passed through on the journey of growing up than the manifestation of a disease that she carried in her biochemistry. The upset in her family had been getting in the way of her development and had been slowing her down. And yes, her brain circuitry probably looked different while she was experiencing stress at home. Removing the stressors of a chaotic home environment and her parents' unhappy marriage allowed Rachel to resume growing normally.

I don't want to make this sound easy, because working with Rachel's parents was anything but. In fact, they were one of the most difficult cases I've ever had. Eileen constantly undermined my credibility and questioned whether family therapy could actually help. In almost every session, Jack said he was on the verge of leaving the marriage. On more than one occasion, when a month went by without my hearing from them, I assumed Jack and Eileen would not be returning to therapy. But they did keep coming back. They felt they had no other choice, because the alternative of giving their daughter an antipsychotic drug was out of the question.

I have told Rachel's story not simply to draw a comparison between drug therapy and family therapy, but also because the story illustrates a broad societal trend. Parents are becoming aware that they need to find out more about the medications that are prescribed for their children. Jack and Eileen were able to evaluate the medications critically, and they felt comfortable with the stimulant drugs. But when it came to giving Rachel an adult antipsychotic like Risperdal, they balked. And that's when they sought alternatives.

I want to state clearly that I do not blame parents who choose to try out medication for a child who has been diagnosed with ADHD. After all, they do so only after a pediatrician or child psychiatrist has told them the medication will help. The doctor, too, is doing what he believes to be best. If the doctor had recommended instead that they make changes in their parenting style or in their daughter's diet, Jack and Eileen would undoubtedly have followed that advice instead. In giving Rachel stimulant drugs for an ADHD diagnosis, her parents were only relying on the advice of trusted professionals.

In turn, the psychiatrist who prescribed Risperdal was relying on what he believed was solid scientific evidence of the drug's efficacy and safety, as well as the reliability of the ADHD diagnosis. However, despite good intentions, the latest twist in the ADHD epidemic in the United States—the prescribing of antipsychotic drugs "off label" to kids when stimulants don't help them—is nothing less than a scandal. Not only are antipsychotic drugs not approved by the FDA for ADHD in children, they carry serious health risks: significant weight gain and an increase of fats in the blood that can lead to cardiovascular problems. Even more worrisome, taking antipsychotics can triple a child's risk of developing type 2 diabetes. Nonetheless, according to a Columbia University study, antipsychotic prescriptions for kids' behavior problems have increased more than sevenfold in the decade of the 2000s (2005 to 2009) as compared to the decade of the 1990s (1993 to 1998). Many of the prescriptions were written by primary care doctors rather than psychiatrists. Today almost one million children in the United States are taking adult antipsychotics like Risperdal, Seroquel, and Abilify.

Laufer's Experiments

The first experiments with antipsychotic drugs for the treatment of hyperactivity in children took place in the 1950s. In 1952, chlorpromazine, widely known by its brand name, Thorazine, was first introduced for treating schizophrenia. The drug was also used to calm agitated patients suffering from severe depression. Surprisingly, researchers also experimented with Thorazine as a means of reducing hyperactivity in children. Pediatrician Maurice Laufer, Charles Bradley's successor as director of the Emma Pendleton Home, with co-authors Eric Denhoff and Gerald Solomons, wrote a paper called "Hyperkinetic Impulse Disorder in Children's Behavior Problems." They found that like amphetamines, Thorazine had a "favorable effect" on hyperkinetic children. Chlorpromazine calmed jumpy children down and enhanced their ability to learn.

Although Laufer was interested in theories that posited neurochemical causes of hyperkinesis—for example, dysfunction of the hypothalamus or of the diencephalon—he believed that parenting was at least one causative factor in hyperkinetic impulse disorder. He thought a disruption in the parents' relationship with each other or emotional problems in one or both parents could cause emotional disturbance in children. He also proposed that overactive kids might need more attentive parenting than children blessed with calmer temperaments. An inexperienced mother, Laufer said, may feel inadequate if her son or daughter does not meet the socially acceptable standard of the quiet, well-behaved child. In this kind of situation, an insecure mother may even develop hostility toward her child because the child reflects badly on her. This hostility can in turn set off a secondary emotional disturbance in the child.

Teachers, too, can be the source of emotional troubles in children. Laufer noted that in the "crowded classrooms" of his day (1956), a teacher might become hostile toward a child who could not sit still, keep his mind on his work, or complete a task, despite having high intelligence. The child, in turn, picks up on his teacher's hostility. This puts even more stress on him, which is compounded by his "unhappy situation at home." The net result is extreme unhappiness in the child, who subsequently develops a distorted and unfavorable image of himself. His behavior can then become even worse.

Laufer's most important insight for our medicalized era is that a thorough understanding of the contribution of the child's home environment, along with both neurological and psychological factors, must be considered in understanding children's disturbed behavior. Even when amphetamines are used, Laufer insisted, "a definite part of the treatment consists of work with the parents." It is crucial, he continued, "not to allow the parents to place sole emphasis upon an organic factor as a means of dismissing any responsibility for making changes in the situation."

The history of child psychiatry after the 1950s was destined, however, to take a different course from the one Laufer advocated. As psychiatry turned toward assuming biological causes for childhood problems, doctors let parents off the hook. But many parents, like Jack and Eileen, are willing to be part of the treatment of their child's ADHD if they think it will be effective, if they are confident that they will not be blamed, and if they can afford it.

Making Informed Choices

Parents have the right—some might say the responsibility—to make informed decisions about which medications are safe or unsafe for their child, just as Jack and Eileen did. And all parents should be given the facts about the psychiatric drugs that are prescribed for their children. Unfortunately, doctors are often pressed for time and are not always forthcoming, or even well informed, about exactly what the drugs are and what the side effects might be. This means that parents need to shoulder the responsibility for researching psychiatric medications and searching for alternatives.

"Addies"

Parents need to be especially vigilant about their teenagers or college-age kids using stimulant drugs. Stimulants' power of cognitive enhancement is making them popular across college campuses nationwide. Today, 25 to 35 percent of American college students abuse ADHD medications, which they call "study drugs," or "academic steroids." In the face of ruthless competition on college campuses, the drugs enhance students' performance by allowing them to go without sleep while cramming for exams. "Everyone else is taking 'addies,'" say college students, "so we have to take them too—or fall behind." Taking stimulants has become socially acceptable because of heightened academic pressure. Most students take the medications orally, but others crush and "snort" them to get an immediate "rush" or "high." This brings these drugs back to their original abuse as a street drug called "speed."

How should we view drugs that alter performance in a society that embraces competitiveness and at the same time condemns the use of steroids to increase natural ability in athletic competitions? Society frowns on using physical steroids in sports but smiles on the use of mental steroids to enhance children's learning. Some colleges and universities, however, have decided that mental steroids are as much a form of cheating as steroids used by athletes. According to the magazine *Campus Safety*, Duke University recently declared that the non-medical use of ADHD medications like Adderall constitutes a form of cheating and violates the school's honor code. George Mason University forbids college clinicians from diagnosing ADHD at all, and the College of William and Mary prohibits college clinicians from prescribing ADHD medications. Other colleges, including Fresno State University and the University of Alabama, require students who bring ADHD medications to campus to sign a contract that they will not give or sell their drugs to other students.

The need for parents to search out alternatives to ADHD medications is all the more pressing as new research is beginning to show that drugs like Ritalin can adversely affect children's brains, impacting their ability to plan ahead, switch between tasks, and be flexible. A 2014 study published in *Frontiers in Neuroscience* found that stimulant drugs have "deeply concerning" effects on the function and plasticity of young people's prefrontal cortex. This study, conducted by researchers at the University of Delaware and Drexel University College of Medicine, calls for more investigation of the effects of stimulants on the cellular and molecular makeup of young people's brains. The study concludes: "Cognitive enhancement is no longer a scientific fiction; we must consider the unique dynamics of the developing brain and proceed cautiously until thorough safety and efficacy parameters have been established."

Policies That Help Children and Parents

While parents can certainly make individual choices in order to protect their kids from overdiagnosis and taking powerful pharmaceuticals, more needs to be done to stop the ADHD epidemic. Policy makers should consider programs in which social workers or pediatric nurses visit the homes of children with behavioral and learning problems to teach parents good parenting skills and evaluate interventions to help children at risk. A federal preschool program, if it comes about, should emulate Finland's model and screen for signs of difficulties in the child's home life early on, before the child enters kindergarten. Parent-training classes should be required for parents of preschoolers at risk for a diagnosis of ADHD. Preschools should not impose academic testing or academic pressure on young children. Scores on standardized tests should not be tied to school funding.

The measures I propose would require profound changes in our society, and they would take time to implement. But with the number of children diagnosed and medicated for ADHD reaching crisis proportions, these measures are absolutely necessary. We are failing millions of children in the United States and we are setting a bad example for the rest of the world. As if it were contagious, ADHD has gained footholds around the globe in countries that rely on the *DSM-5* and American psychiatry.

There are, however, some signs of hope. Schools are becoming aware of how adverse childhood experiences affect children's ability to concentrate and behave in the classroom and are devising individualized interventions for children who need help. Many schools are willing to make accommodations for children like Ricky who need opportunities to leave their desks and move around during the school day. Pediatricians are becoming aware of how family issues impact children, and they are willing to recommend family interventions before prescribing stimulant medications.

A cultural shift away from medicating children is daunting in the face of Big Pharma and the established medical order. But these institutions exist and serve only at the pleasure of the public. We owe our children protection from the self-serving motives of these powerful institutions. We rely on the strength of healthy families led by thoughtful and well-informed parents to make decisions that are in the best interests of their children. And to make good decisions, parents need to be attuned to their kids.

If you are a parent who suspects your child has ADHD, I recommend you make a point of listening to your child carefully to find out what is amiss in his world. Turn off your cell phone (or leave it in another room) and give your child your full attention. If your child is jumpy and fidgety or if he is underperforming at school, it's best not to jump to a hasty conclusion that there is a medical explanation for these behaviors. As I have suggested in this book, medical metaphors for childhood behaviors are unique to our culture and era. What's really important is for you to listen to your child's feelings and acknowledge them. The more you understand your child's feelings, the more you will understand his behavior. For example, if your child says "I hate school," instead of lecturing him on the importance of education, try to be empathic. Say something like "It must be difficult to sit still all day" or "I understand that you're feeling frustrated with school right now." Don't try to fix the problem right away or ask your child a lot of questions. Take time simply to listen and reflect back your child's feeling. Therapists call this "reflective listening" and it's one of the oldest and most effective techniques in the therapist's toolbox.

At times, all of us just want to vent our feelings and feel heard. In these moments we don't want someone to fix the situation or give us advice on how we could fix it ourselves. We just want someone to listen and understand how we are feeling. Kids are the same. As much as parents want to find quick solutions to their children's problems, the first step to helping a troubled child is to listen and understand what the child is truly feeling.

Listening might not always be easy—for example, if your husband is a devoted soccer fan and your son goofs off on the soccer field and tells you he hates soccer. It was not easy for one mother to hear her daughter say that she didn't like her new teacher at the beginning of the school year. Having heard great things about this particular teacher, the mother hastily pointed out the teacher's many good qualities instead of simply hearing her daughter's feeling. When I mentioned this to her, she realized that her daughter needed more understanding and acceptance. Listening to and validating a daughter's feeling doesn't mean that a mother should rush out and change her daughter's classroom. It means only that she accepts and understands her child's feeling in the moment. If you listen to your child and acknowledge her feelings (whether you agree with them or not), your child will feel like you really care about her and understand her. When parents really listen to their child, the child will start to feel happier inside and in time his behavior will improve as well.

ACKNOWLEDGMENTS

It truly takes a village to write a book, and I feel blessed in having a caring and supportive village that sustained me throughout the writing process. First, my gratitude goes to my husband and soul mate, Gene, who read and critiqued every draft of every chapter with a scientific eagle eye. The book benefits immeasurably from his feedback. I thank Lauren Marino, my inspiring editor at Avery, for her wise editorial guidance and for her enthusiasm for this project from the beginning. I thank Brooke Carey at Avery for her elegant and meticulous sculpting of the final manuscript. Her sage queries and suggestions were a significant contribution. My thanks go also to Lauren's assistant, Emily Wunderlich, for her comments on an early draft of Chapter 4. I thank Linda Carbone for her editorial help in the book's early stages and Jo Ann Miller for her editorial wisdom throughout. Thanks go to Nellys Liang for her inspired cover design. My gratitude goes to Karen Mayer for her sage advice and her subtle sense of language. I thank Muriel Jorgensen for her meticulous and insightful copy editing.

Many people helped me with this book in various ways. I thank

Manuel Vallée for sending me his important research and for sharing the work of his colleagues. I thank Dr. Bruno Harlé for his generous collegiality and his insights about ADHD in France. I thank my sons, Dan and Jay, for helping me understand the media milieu of the millennial generation. I thank all my clan for their ongoing love and support: Dan, Ellie, Teddy, Huck, Monty, Jessica, Jay, and Hayley. I thank Stuart Kaplan, Susan Parry, Matt Healy, and Katie King for various kinds of support and help. I thank my clients who have taught me so much over the past twenty-five years. I am extremely grateful to readers of *Pills Are Not for Preschoolers* and "Why French Kids Don't Have ADHD" who wrote to me with their stories, questions, and words of encouragement. I thank my early mentors, true giants in their fields, psychiatrist Jarl Dyrud and family therapist Jay Haley.

I thank my literary agent and the guardian angel of this book, Susan Lee Cohen.

NOTES

· · · · · ·

Introduction: A Season in Childhood

xv *Centers for Disease Control and Prevention data*: Craig Garfield et al., "Trends in Attention Deficit Hyperactivity Disorder Ambulatory Diagnosis and Medical Treatment in the United States 2000–2010," *American Pediatrics* 12, no. 2 (2012): 110–16.

xviii *with psychotherapy or family counseling*: Manuel Vallée, "Resisting American Psychiatry: French Opposition to DSM-III, Biological Reductionism and the Pharmaceutical Ethos," *Advances in Medical Sociology* 12 (2011): 85–110.

Chapter 1: What Is ADHD?

8 *After the publication of the* DSM-III-R: "ADHD: The Diagnostic Criteria," *Frontline*, 2014, http://www.pbs.org/wgbh/pages/frontline/shows/medicating/adhd/diagnostic.html.

12 *became comfortable with taking amphetamines*: Alan Schwarz, "Risky Rise of the Good-Grade Pill," *New York Times*, June 9, 2012.

Chapter 2: A Tale of Many Cultures

22 *taking psychostimulants has increased*: Michel Lecendreux et al., "Prevalence of Attention Deficit Disorder and Associated Features Among Children in France," *Journal of Attention Disorders* 15, no. 6 (2011): 516–24.

22 *according to a recent Pharma-funded telephone survey*: Ibid., 516, originally published online August 2, 2010.

23 *looked for a social environment cause*: The CFTMEA encourages psychiatrists to identify "factors related to the environment" such as "emotional, educational, social and cultural deficiencies, as well as bad treatments and negligence." Vallée, "Resisting American Psychiatry."

23 *French child psychiatry's developmental approach*: Ibid.

26 *"diagnoses into other systems"*: Pierre Pichot, "The French Approach to Psychiatric Classification," *British Journal of Psychiatry* 144 (1984): 113–18.

26 *updated in later editions*: Ibid.

27 *"therapeutic attention on isolated symp-*

toms": Roger Misès, "French Classification for Child and Adolescent Mental Disorders," *Psychopathology* 35 (2002): 176–80.

27 *CFTMEA explicitly discourages giving a child*: Vallée, "Resisting American Psychiatry."

28 *into the language of everyday life*: Sherry Turkle, *Psychoanalytic Politics: Jacques Lacan and Freud's French Revolution* (New York: Guilford Press, 1992).

28 *even more than Americans*: A. Dorozynski, "France Tackles Psychotropic Drug Problem," *British Journal of Medicine* 312 (1996): 997.

28 *adults took antidepressants*: Bill Chappell, "Third of French Are on Psychoactive Drugs, Agency Says," National Public Radio, *The Two-Way*, May 20, 2014.

28 *her smiling child holding a paper with a B+ on it*: Alan Schwarz, "The Selling of Attention Deficit Disorder," *New York Times*, December 14, 2013.

29 *fewer children qualify for the diagnosis*: M. Dopfner et al., "How Often Do Children Meet ICD-10/DSM-IV Criteria of Attention Deficit-/Hyperactivity Disorder and Hyperkinetic Disorder?," *European Child and Adolescent Psychiatry* 17 (December 2008): Suppl. 1:5–9–70.

31 *"personality disorder" and "learning disability"*: Giovanni Frazzetto et al., "'I Bambini e le Droghe': The Right to Ritalin vs. the Right to Childhood in Italy," *Biosocieties* 2 (2007): 393–412.

31 *to be on a continuum with normal childhood behaviors*: Ibid.

32 *provide them with a firm cadre*: Pamela Druckerman, *Bringing Up Bébé* (New York: Penguin, 2012).

32 *sociologists Claude Fischler and Estelle Masson*: "France, Europe, the United States: What Eating Means to Us: Interview with Claude Fischler and Estelle Masson," Lemangeur-ocha.com, posted online January 16, 2008.

33 *refuse to eat, as many American children do*: Jacob Azerrad and Paul Chance, "Why Our Kids Are out of Control," *Psychology Today*, September 1, 2001.

34 *correlate with a child being diagnosed with ADHD*: Anders Hjern et al., "Social Adversity Predicts ADHD-Medication in School Children—a National Cohort Study," *Acta Paediatrica* 99, no. 6 (June 2010): 920–24.

34 *Substantial research*: Carolyn Webster-Stratton and Mary Hammond, "Treating Children with Early-Onset Conduct Problems: A Comparison of Child and Parent Training Interventions," *Journal of Consulting and Clinical Psychology* 65, no. 1 (1997): 93–109.

36 *without taking medication*: Benedict Carey, "Parenting as Therapy for Child's Mental Disorders," *New York Times*, December 22, 2006.

Chapter 3: How a Diagnosis Became an Epidemic

45 *Philip Ash had published a study*: Alix Spiegel, "The Dictionary of Disorder: How One Man Revolutionized Psychiatry," *New Yorker*, January 3, 2005.

46 *declined by 16 percent*: Vallée, "Resisting American Psychiatry."

46 *upsetting life situations*: Hannah Decker, "How Kraepelinian Was Kraepelin? How Kraepelinian Are the Neo-Kraepelinians?—From Emil Kraepelin to the DSM-III," *History of Psychiatry* 18, no. 3 (2007): 337–60.

46 *Eli Robins, Samuel Guze, and George Winokur*: Medical sociologist Manuel Vallée

first made me aware of the key role of the Washington University trio, Robins, Guze, and Winokur, in creating the biological model of psychiatry and influencing the *DSM-III*.

48 *"not soon be put down"*: Hannah Decker, *The Making of DSM-III: A Diagnostic Manual's Conquest of American Psychiatry* (Oxford: Oxford University Press, 2013).

49 *"sit at the feet" of Eli Robins*: Ibid.

49 *specific plans for the new DSM*: Ibid.

51 *developers of PRIME-MD*: Herb Kutchins and Stuart Kirk, *Making Us Crazy* (New York: Free Press, 1997), 13.

53 *"interrelationships are clearly the problem"*: Ibid., 260.

53 *"our decisions was pretty modest"*: Spiegel, "The Dictionary of Disorder."

53 *among the group of authors*: Decker, *The Making of DSM-III*.

53 *"result of specific research data"*: James Davies, *Cracked: The Unhappy Truth About Psychiatry* (London: Pegasus, 2014).

54 *Spitzer later admitted in an interview*: Ibid.

54 *was decided by a vote*: Ibid.

58 *benefits of psychiatric drugs*: Gardiner Harris and Benedict Carey, "Researchers Fail to Reveal Full Drug Pay," *New York Times*, June 8, 2008.

58 *benefited drug industry products*: Gardiner Harris, "Drug Makers Are Advocacy Group's Biggest Donors," *New York Times*, October 21, 2009.

59 *influence on medical practice*: Ibid.

59 *"parent-child relationship"*: Dorothy Bloch, *So the Witch Won't Eat Me: Fantasy and the Child's Fear of Infanticide* (New York: Grove Press, 1978).

59 *congenital, incurable illness*: Ibid.

59 *mirroring, understanding, and sympathy*: Alice Miller, *The Drama of the Gifted Child* (New York: Basic Books, 1997).

60 *wiring of children's brains*: Bruce Perry, *The Boy Who Was Raised as a Dog* (New York: Perseus, 2006).

61 *experience by age eighteen*: Ibid.

62 *mere twenty-minute interview*: Alan Schwarz, "Drowned in a Stream of Prescriptions," *New York Times*, February 2, 2013.

63 *More than half*: Lisa Cosgrove et al., "Financial Ties Between *DSM-IV* Panel Members and the Pharmaceutical Industry," *Psychotherapy and Psychosomatics* 75, no. 3 (2006): 154–60.

Chapter 4: Big Pharma and Biological Psychiatry

66 *"could benefit from Ritalin"*: Gina Kolata, "Boom in Ritalin Sales Raises Ethical Issues," *New York Times*, May 15, 1996.

66 *paid to them by drug companies*: Harris and Carey, "Researchers Fail to Reveal Full Drug Pay."

67 *"psychopharmacology maven for ADHD"*: Schwarz, "The Selling of Attention Deficit Disorder."

73 *"audience of healthy schoolchildren"*: Madeleine Strohl, "Bradley's Benzedrine Studies on Children with Behavioral Disorders," *Yale Journal of Biology and Medicine* 84, no. 1 (March 2011): 27–33.

73 *giving amphetamines to students for performance enhancement*: Ibid.

74 *In 1902, the British physician George Still*: George Still, "Some Abnormal Physical Conditions in Children," *Lancet*, 1. (1902); 1008–1012.

75 *diagnosed with ADHD*: Judith Rapoport et al., "Dextroamphetamine: Cognitive

and Behavioral Effects in Normal Prepubertal Boys," *Science* 199, no. 4328 (February 3, 1978): 560–63.

75 *college students take prescription stimulants illicitly*: Alan Schwarz, "Attention Deficit Drugs Face New Campus Rules," *New York Times*, April 30, 2014.

78 *questionable drug company practices*: Morton Mintz, *The Therapeutic Nightmare* (New York: Houghton Mifflin, 1965).

78 *Haskell Weinstein, testified before the subcommittee*: Ibid.

78 *"and rarely is publication refused"*: Ibid.

78 *once-a-day medicine for ADHD*: Melody Petersen, "Madison Ave. Has Growing Role in the Business of Drug Research," *New York Times*, November 22, 2002.

79 *longer-acting form of Ritalin*: Linda Logdberg, "Being the Ghost in the Machine: A Medical Ghostwriter's Personal View," *Public Library of Science, Medicine* 8, no. 8 (August 9, 2011).

79 *Logdberg disagreed*: Ibid.

79 *"take steps to prevent it"*: Petersen, "Madison Ave. Has Growing Role."

80 *Forest products is discussed*: Ibid.

80 *for journal advertisements*: Robert Whitaker, *Anatomy of an Epidemic* (New York: Crown, 2010).

80 *in medical journals overall*: Adriane Fugh-Berman et al., "Advertising in Medical Journals: Should Current Practices Change?" *Public Library of Science, Medicine* 3, no. 7: e303. doi: 10.1371/journal.pmed.0030303.

81 *"improved for children's use"*: Roni Caryn Rabin, "Drugs to treat A.D.H.D. Reach the Preschool Set," *New York Times*, October 24, 2011.

82 *American Academy of Pediatrics*: Evelyn Pringle, "The Case of the Vaccination Profiteers," *Public Record*, November 5, 2010.

82 *was never mentioned*: Larry Silver, "Attention Deficit-Hyperactivity Disorder and Learning Disabilities Booklet for the Classroom Teacher," Ciba-Geigy, 1990.

84 *"baited" by Ciba-Geigy*: Alan Schwarz and Sarah Cohen, "ADHD Seen in 11% of U.S. Children as Diagnoses Rise," *New York Times*, March 31, 2013.

84 *by child psychiatrist Harvey Parker*: Frontline, http://www.pbs.org/wgbh/pages/frontline/shows/medicating/interviews/parker.html.

84 *child's brain more "normal"*: Whitaker, *Anatomy of an Epidemic*.

85 *"preparation in the United States"*: "Use of Methylphenidate for the Treatment of Attention Deficit Disorder," *Report of the United Nations International Narcotics Control Board* (New York: United Nations, 1995), 20–22.

87 *unwilling to test the case in court*: Karin Klein, "Pencils, Pens, Meds," *Los Angeles Times*, August 20, 2007.

87 *"Give me the grape"*: Ibid.

88 *the number of prescriptions*: Ibid.

88 *"how the world is changing"*: Olga Khazan, "How Supportive Parenting Protects the Brain," *Atlantic*, June 26, 2014.

88 *"officials in an effort to lift drug sales"*: Katie Thomas, "Glaxo Says It Will Stop Paying Doctors to Promote Drugs," *New York Times*, December 16, 2013.

89 *he will stop saying so*: Schwarz and Cohen, "ADHD Seen in 11% of U.S. Children."

89 *kids using stimulants as "mental steroids"*: Ibid.

91 *power of stimulant medications*: Mintz, *The Therapeutic Nightmare*.

92 *the Individuals with Disabilities Education Act*: Frontline Report: "Federal Laws Pertaining to ADHD Diagnosed Children," 2001, www.pbs.org/wgbh/pages/front

line/shows/medicating/schools/feds
.html.

92 *leading category of disability in children*:
Whitaker, *Anatomy of an Epidemic*.

Chapter 5: The Message in the Media

104 *from one form to another*: John P. Ioannidis, "Why Most Research Findings Are
False," *Public Library of Science, Medicine* 2, no. 8 (August 2005).

106 *several members of the Wellcome Trust*:
Wellcome.ac.uk, Organization, Technology Transfer Strategy Panel.

107 *it is widely subject to cultural interpretation*: François Gonon et al., "Misrepresentation of Neuroscience Data Might
Give Rise to Misleading Conclusions in
the Media: The Case of Attention Deficit
Hyperactivity Disorder," *Public Library of
Science* 6, no. 1 (January 2011).

108 *both Stephen V. Faraone and Samuele
Cortese*: Samuele Cortese et al., "Sleep in
Children with Attention-Deficit/Hyper-
activity Disorder: Meta-Analysis of Sub-
jective and Objective Studies," *Journal
of the American Academy of Child and
Adolescent Psychiatry* 48, no. 9, 894–908
(September 2009).

109 *between a dopamine deficit and ADHD*:
François Gonon, "The Dopaminergic
Hypothesis of Attention Deficit Hyper-
activity Disorder Needs Re-examining,"
Trends in Neuroscience 32, no. 1 (2008).

111 *In a remarkable 2012 lecture*: Dorothy
Bishop, Emanuel Miller Memorial Lecture, Association for Child and Adolescent Mental Health, London, March 14,
2012.

Chapter 6: Why American Schools Have to Change

120 *"equalizing instrument for society"*: Jenny
Anderson, "From Finland, an Intriguing

School-Reform Model," *New York Times*,
December 12, 2011.

123 *enhance their learning*: Alfie Kohn, *The
Homework Myth: Why Our Kids Get Too
Much of a Bad Thing* (Cambridge, MA: Da
Capo Press, 2006).

127 *in the* Journal of Health Economics: San-
ford Newmark, "Are ADHD Medications
Overprescribed?," *Wall Street Journal*,
February 14, 2013.

127 *same grade in school*: Todd E. Elder, "The
Importance of Relative Standards in
ADHD Diagnoses: Evidence Based on
Exact Birth Dates," *Journal of Health
Economics* 29, no. 5 (September 2010):
641–56.

128 *throughout their school years*: "Younger
Children in the Classroom Likely Over-
diagnosed with ADHD: UBC Research,"
University of British Columbia media
release, March 5, 2012, http://www
.publicaffairs.ubc.ca/2012/03/05/.

130 *in* Pediatrics *in 2012*: Jack P. Shonkoff
and Andrew S. Garner, "The Lifelong
Effects of Early Childhood Adversity and
Toxic Stress," *Pediatrics*, December 26,
2011.

134 *to return to the classroom*: Jane Ellen
Stevens, "Q and A with Suzanne Savall,
Principal of Trauma-Informed Elemen-
tary School in Spokane, WA," Aces Too
High, August 20, 2013, http://acestoo
high.com/.

136 *"Someone would have told me in medi-
cal school"*: Jane Ellen Stevens, "The
Adverse Childhood Experiences Study:
The Largest Public Health Study You
Never Heard Of," *Huffington Post*, Octo-
ber 8, 2012.

137 *addressed the issue of toxic stress*: Schon-
koff and Garner, "The Lifelong Effects of
Early Childhood Adversity."

137 *childhood adversity and toxic stress*: Ibid.

145 *California was one of the last*: Maggie Koerth-Baker, "The Not-So-Hidden Cause Behind the ADHD Epidemic," *New York Times*, October 15, 2013.

146 *"relationship between parent and child"*: Alice Charach et al., "Interventions for Preschool Children at High Risk for ADHD: A Comparative Effectiveness Review," *Pediatrics*, April 1, 2013.

146 *children in Kansas and Missouri*: David Bornstein, "Teaching Children to Calm Themselves," *New York Times*, March 19, 2014.

Chapter 7: Let Food Be Thy Medicine

151 *medical journals, such as* Ecology of Disease *and* Delaware Medical Journal: Matthew Smith, *An Alternative History of Hyperactivity: Food Additives and the Feingold Diet* (New Brunswick, NJ: Rutgers University Press, 2011).

161 *at least in some children*: Newmark, "Are ADHD Medications Overprescribed?"

162 *2004 article in* Pediatrics: Nathaniel Zelnik et al., "Range of Neurological Disorders on Patients with Celiac Disease," *Pediatrics* 113, no. 6 (June 6, 2004).

Chapter 9: Time-Tested Tactics for Good Parenting

199 *negative impact on children's psychological development*: Gordon Harold et al., *Not in Front of the Children? How Conflict Between Parents Affects Children.* (London: OnePlusOne Marriage and Partnership Research, 2001).

201 *after their baby is born*: Pamela Druckerman, *Bébé Day by Day* (New York: Penguin, 2013).

211 *A 2013 study by researchers at the University of Illinois*: Gretchen Reynolds, "Put the Physical in Education," *New York Times*, September 4, 2014.

211 *Ratey believes that physical activity*: James Hamblin, "Exercise Is ADHD Medication," *Atlantic*, September 29, 2014.

Chapter 10: Protecting Children in the Age of Adderall

212 *the battle cry of "retreat"*: Hannah Rosin, "The Overprotected Kid," *Atlantic*, March 19, 2014.

221 *risk of developing type 2 diabetes*: Carole Bartoo, "Antipsychotic Drug Use in Children for Mood/Behavior Disorders Increases Type 2 Diabetes Risk," *Research News@Vanderbilt*, August 22, 2013, Vanderbilt University.

221 *rather than psychiatrists*: M. Olfson et al., "National Trends in the Office-Based Treatment of Children, Adolescents and Adults with Antipsychotics," *JAMA Psychiatry* 69, no. 12 (December 2012).

222 *set off a secondary emotional disturbance in the child*: Maurice Laufer and Eric Denhoff, "Hyperkinetic Impulse Disorder in Children's Behavior Problems," *Journal of Pediatrics* 50 (1957): 463–74.

BIBLIOGRAPHY

Acquaviva, Eric. "Psychotropic Medication in the French Child and Adolescent Population: Prevalence Estimation from Health Insurance Data and National Self-Report Survey Data." *BMC Psychiatry* 9 (2009): 72.

"ADHD: The Diagnostic Criteria." *Frontline*, 2014, http://www.pbs.org/wgbh/pages/frontline/shows/medicating/adhd/diagnostic.html.

Anderson, Jenny. "From Finland, an Intriguing School-Reform Model." *New York Times*, December 12, 2011.

Azerrad, J., and Paul Chance. "Why Our Kids Are Out of Control," *Psychology Today*, September 1, 2001.

Bartoo, Carole. "Antipsychotic Drug Use in Children for Mood/Behavior Disorders Increases Type 2 Diabetes Risk." *Research News@Vanderbilt*, August 22, 2013, Vanderbilt University. https://medschool.vanderbilt.edu/psychiatry/news.

"Beautiful Minds: Medicating America's Children." *Economist*, March 1, 2014.

Bishop, Dorothy. Emanuel Miller Memorial Lecture. Association for Child and Adolescent Mental Health, March 14, 2012.

Bloch, Dorothy. *So the Witch Won't Eat Me: Fantasy and the Child's Fear of Infanticide.* New York: Grove Press, 1978.

Bornstein, David. "Protecting Children from Toxic Stress." *New York Times*, October 30, 2013.

———. "Teaching Children to Calm Themselves." *New York Times*, March 19, 2014.

Bradley, Charles. "The Behavior of Children Receiving Benzedrine." *American Journal of Psychiatry* 94 (1937): 577–81.

Bradley, Charles, and Margaret Bowen. "Amphetamine (Benzedrine) Therapy of Children's Behavior Disorders." *American Journal of Orthopsychiatry* 11 (1940): 92–103.

Braithwaite, John. *Corporate Crime in the Pharmaceutical Industry.* London: Routledge and Kegan Paul, 1984.

Breggin, Peter. *Talking Back to Ritalin*. New York: Da Capo Press, 1997.

Carey, Benedict. "Parenting as Therapy for Child's Mental Disorders." *New York Times*, December 22, 2006.

Chappell, Bill. "Third of French Are on Psychoactive Drugs, Agency Says." National Public Radio, *The Two-Way*, May 20, 2014.

Charach, Alice, et al. "Interventions for Preschool Children at High Risk for ADHD: A Comparative Effectiveness Review." *Pediatrics*, April 1, 2013.

Cortese, Samuele, et al. "Sleep in Children with Attention-Deficit/Hyperactivity Disorder: Meta-Analysis of Subjective and Objective Studies." *Journal of the American Academy of Child and Adolescent Psychiatry* 48, no. 12 (September 2009): 894–908.

———. "Misunderstandings of the Genetics and Neurobiology of ADHD: Moving Beyond Anachronisms." *American Journal of Human Genetics, Part B*, August 2011.

———. "What Should Be Said to the Lay Public Regarding ADHD Etiology Based on Unbiased Systematic Qualitative Evidence?" *American Journal of Human Genetics*, August 2011.

Cosgrove, Lisa, et al. "Financial Ties Between DSM-IV Panel Members and the Pharmaceutical Industry." *Psychotherapy and Psychosomatics* 75, no. 3 (2006): 154–60.

D'Andrea, Wendy, et al. "Understanding Interpersonal Trauma in Children: Why We Need a Developmentally Appropriate Trauma Diagnosis." *American Journal of Orthopsychiatry* 82, no. 2 (2012): 187–200.

Davies, James. *Cracked: The Unhappy Truth About Psychiatry*. London: Pegasus, 2014.

Decker, Hannah. "How Kraepelinian Was Kraepelin? How Kraepelinian Are the Neo-Kraepelinians?—From Emil Kraepelin to the *DSM-III*." *History of Psychiatry* 18, no. 3 (2007): 337–60.

———. *The Making of DSM-III, a Diagnostic Manual's Conquest of American Psychiatry*. Oxford: Oxford University Press, 2013.

Dopfner, M., et al. "How Often Do Children Meet ICD-10/DSM-IV Criteria of Attention Deficit-/Hyperactivity Disorder and Hyperkinetic Disorder?" *European Child and Adolescent Psychiatry* 17 (December 2008): Suppl. 1:59–70.

Dorozynski, A. "France Tackles Psychotropic Drug Problem." *British Journal of Medicine* 312 (1996): 997.

Druckerman, Pamela. *Bébé Day by Day*. New York: Penguin, 2013.

———. *Bringing Up Bébé*. New York: Penguin, 2012.

Elder, Todd E. "The Importance of Relative Standards in ADHD Diagnoses: Evidence Based on Exact Birth Dates." *Journal of Health Economics* 29, no. 5 (September 2010): 641–56.

Feingold, Benjamin. "Hyperkinesis and Learning Disabilities Linked to the Ingestion of Artificial Food Colors and Flavors." *American Journal of Nursing* 5 (May 1975): 797–803.

Foucault, Michel. *Madness and Civilization*. New York: Vintage, 1965.

———. *The Order of Things: An Archeology of the Human Sciences*. New York: Random House, 1970.

"France, Europe, the United States: What Eating Means to Us: Interview with Claude Fischler and Estelle Masson." Lemangeurocha.com, posted online January 16, 2008.

Frazzetto, Giovanni, et al. "'I Bambini e le Droghe': The Right to Ritalin vs. the Right to Childhood in Italy." *Biosocieties* 2 (2007): 393–412.

Freedman, David. "Lies, Damned Lies, and Medical Science." *Atlantic*, November 2010.

Fugh-Berman, Adriane. "Advertising in Medical Journals: Should Current Practices Change?" *Public Library of Science, Medicine* 3, no. 7: e303. doi: 10.1371/journal .pmed.0030303.

Garfield, Craig, et al. "Trends in Attention Deficit Hyperactivity Disorder Ambulatory Diagnosis and Medical Treatment in the United States 2000–2010." *American Pediatrics* 12, no. 2 (2012): 110–16.

Garner, Andrew, and Jack Shonkoff. "Early Childhood Adversity, Toxic Stress, and the Role of the Pediatrician: Translating Developmental Science into Lifelong Health." *Pediatrics*, December 26, 2011.

Gold, Mark, et al. "Adolescent Abuse of ADHD Medications: A Sad Truth." *Pediatrics*, Letter to the Editor, September 11, 2009.

Goleman, Daniel. "Push Is On for Family Doctors to Spot Psychiatric Problems." *New York Times*, December 14, 1994.

Gonon, François. "The Dopaminergic Hypothesis of Attention-Deficit/Hyperactivity Disorder Needs Re-examining." *Trends in Neuroscience* 32, no. 1 (2008).

Gonon, François, et al. "Misrepresentation of Neuroscience Data Might Give Rise to Misleading Conclusions in the Media: The Case of Attention Deficit Hyperactivity Disorder." *Public Library of Science* 6, no. 1 (January 2011).

Hamblin, James. "Exercise Is ADHD Medication." *Atlantic*, September 29, 2014.

Harold, Gordon, et al. *Not in Front of the Children? How Conflict Between Parents Affects Children*. London: OnePlusOne Marriage and Partnership Research, 2001.

Harris, Gardiner. "Drug Makers Are Advocacy Group's Biggest Donors." *New York Times*, October 21, 2009.

Harris, Gardiner, and Benedict Carey. "Researchers Fail to Reveal Full Drug Pay." *New York Times*, June 8, 2008.

Healy, Melissa. "Growing Up with, and Out of, ADHD." *New York Times*, January 28, 2008.

Hjern, Anders, et al. "Social Adversity Predicts ADHD-Medication in School Children—A National Cohort Study." *Acta Paediatrica* 99, no. 6 (June 2010): 920–24.

House of Representatives of the United States. *Federal Involvement in the Use of Behavior Modification Drugs on Grammar School Children on the Right to Privacy Issue*. Washington, DC: US Government Printing Office, 1970.

Hruska, Bronwen. "Raising the Ritalin Generation." *New York Times*, August 18, 2012.

Ioannidis, John. "Why Most Research Findings Are False." *Public Library of Science, Medicine* 2, no. 8 (August 2005).

Jenner, F., and A. Monteiro. Letter to the Editor. *Schizophrenia Bulletin*, 1982.

"Journalistic Deficit Disorder: What Newspapers Don't Say Matters as Much as What They Do." *Economist*, September 22, 2012.

Jutel, Annemarie. "Sociology of Diagnosis: A Preliminary Review." *Sociology of Health and Illness* 31, no. 2 (2009): 278–99.

Khazan, Olga. "How Supportive Parenting Protects the Brain." *Atlantic*, June 26, 2014.

Klein, Karin. "Pencils, Pens, Meds." *Los Angeles Times*, August 20, 2007.

Koerth-Baker, Maggie. "The Not-So-Hidden Cause Behind the ADHD Epidemic." *New York Times*, October 15, 2013.

Kohn, Alfie. *The Homework Myth: Why Our Kids Get Too Much of a Bad Thing*. Cambridge, MA: Da Capo Press, 2006.

Kolata, Gina. "Boom in Ritalin Sales Raises Ethical Issues." *New York Times*, May 15, 1996.

Kowalczyk, Liz. "Harvard Doctors Punished over Pay." *Boston Globe*, July 2, 2011.

Kramer, Peter. *Listening to Prozac*. New York: Penguin, 1993.

Kutchins, Herb, and Stuart Kirk. *Making Us Crazy*. New York: Free Press, 1997.

Laufer, Maurice, and Eric Denhoff. "Hyperkinetic Impulse Disorder in Children's Behavior Problems." *Journal of Pediatrics* 50 (1957): 463–74.

Lecendreux, Michel, et al. "Prevalence of Attention Deficit Disorder and Associated Features Among Children in France." *Journal of Attention Disorders* 15, no. 6 (2011): 516–24.

Logdberg, Linda. "Being the Ghost in the Machine: A Medical Ghostwriter's Personal View." *Public Library of Science, Medicine* 8, no. 8 (August 9, 2011).

Marcus, Gary. "Neuroscience Fiction." *New Yorker*, December 2, 2012.

Miller, Alice. *The Drama of the Gifted Child*. New York: Basic Books, 1997.

Mintz, Morton. *The Therapeutic Nightmare*. New York: Houghton Mifflin, 1965.

Misès, Roger, et al. "French Classification for Child and Adolescent Mental Disorders." *Psychopathology* 35 (2002): 176–80.

National Institute of Mental Health. "Director's Blog: Transforming Diagnosis." April 29, 2013. imh.nih.gov/about/director/2013/transforming-diagnosis.shtml.

Newmark, Sanford. "Are ADHD Medications Overprescribed?" *Wall Street Journal*, February 14, 2013.

O'Brien, Carl. "Parenting Courses Help Reduce ADHD Symptoms Among Children, Study Shows." *Irish Times*, November 21, 2013.

O'Leary, KD. "Pills or Skills for Hyperactive children?" *Journal of Applied Behavior Analysis* 133, no. 1 (Spring 1980): 191–204.

Olfson, Mark, et al. "National Trends in the Office-Based Treatment of Children, Adolescents and Adults with Antipsychotics." *JAMA Psychiatry* 69, no. 12 (December 2012).

Parry, Susan. E-mail to the author, August 4, 2014.

Partanen, Anu. "What Americans Keep Ignoring About Finland's School Success." *Atlantic*, December 29, 2011.

Payer, Lynn. *Medicine and Culture*. New York: Henry Holt, 1988.

Perry, Bruce. *The Boy Who Was Raised as a Dog*. New York: Perseus, 2006.

Petersen, Melody. "Madison Ave. Has Growing Role in the Business of Drug Research." *New York Times*, November 22, 2002.

Phelan, Thomas. *1-2-3 Magic*. Glen Ellyn, IL: Parent Magic, 2003.

Phillips, C. "Medicine Goes to School: Teachers as Sickness Brokers for ADHD." *Public Library of Science Medicine*, April 11, 2006.

Pichot, Pierre. "The French Approach to Psychiatric Classification." *British Journal of Psychiatry* 144 (1984): 113–18.

Pringle, Evelyn. "The Case of the Vaccination Profiteers." *Public Record*, November 5, 2010.

Quart, Alissa. "Neuroscience: Under Attack." *New York Times*, November 23, 2012.

Rabin, Roni Caryn. "Drugs to Treat A.D.H.D. Reach the Preschool Set." *New York Times*, October 24, 2011.

Rapoport, Judith, et al. "Dextroamphetamine: Cognitive and Behavioral Effects in Normal Prepubertal Boys." *Science* 199, no. 4328 (February 3, 1978): 560–63.

Resnick, Brian. "The Mess of No Child Left Behind." *Atlantic*, December 16, 2011.

Reynolds, G. "Put the Physical in Education." *New York Times*, September 4, 2014.

Rosin, Hannah. "The Overprotected Kid." *Atlantic*, March 19, 2014.

Ruiz, Rebecca. "Are There Non-medication Alternatives for ADHD Treatment?" Aces TooHigh.com, July 8, 2014.

Russell, Ginny. "The Association of Attention Deficit Hyperactivity Disorder with Socioeconomic Disadvantage: Alternative Explanations and Evidence." *Journal of Child Psychology and Psychiatry* 55, no. 5 (2014): 436–45.

Sahlberg, Pasi. *Finnish Lessons: What the World Can Learn from Educational Change in Finland*. New York: Teachers College Press, 2010.

Schwarz, Alan. "Drowned in a Stream of Prescriptions." *New York Times*, February 2, 2013.

———. "Idea of New Attention Disorder Spurs Research and Debate." *New York Times*, April 11, 2014.

———. "Risky Rise of the Good-Grade Pill." *New York Times*, June 9, 2012.

———. "The Selling of Attention Deficit Disorder." *New York Times*, December 14, 2013.

———. "Thousands of Toddlers Are Medicated for ADHD, Report Finds, Raising Worries." *New York Times*, May 16, 2014.

Schwarz, Alan, and Sarah Cohen. "ADHD Seen in 11% of U.S. Children as Diagnoses Rise." *New York Times*, March 31, 2013.

Setlik, Jennifer, et al. "Adolescent Prescription Medication Abuse Is Rising Along with Prescriptions for These Medications." *Pediatrics* 124 (September 3, 2009).

Shonkoff, Jack, and Andrew Garner. "The Lifelong Effects of Early Childhood Adversity and Toxic Stress." *Pediatrics*, December 26, 2011.

Silver, Larry. "Attention Deficit-Hyperactivity Disorder and Learning Disabilities Booklet for the Classroom Teacher." Ciba-Geigy, 1990.

Singh, Ilina. "Bad Boys, Good Mothers, and the 'Miracle' of Ritalin." *Science in Context* 15, no. 4 (2002): 577–603.

Smith, Matthew. *An Alternative History of Hyperactivity: Food Additives and the Feingold Diet*. New Brunswick, NJ: Rutgers University Press, 2011.

Spiegel, Alix. "The Dictionary of Disorder: How One Man Revolutionized Psychiatry." *New Yorker*, January 3, 2005.

Spitzer, Robert. Letter to the Editor. *Schizophrenia Bulletin* 8 (1982).

Spitzer, R., et al. "Utility of a New Procedure for Diagnosing Mental Disorders in Primary Care." *JAMA* 272, no. 22 (December 14, 1994): 1749–56.

Sroufe, Alan. "Ritalin Gone Wrong." *New York Times*, January 28, 2012.

Stevens, Jane Ellen. "The Adverse Childhood Experiences Study: The Largest Public Health Study You Never Heard Of." *Huffington Post*, October 8, 2012.

———. "Q and A with Suzanne Savall, Principal of Trauma-Informed Elementary School in Spokane, WA." Aces Too High Web site, August 20, 2013. http://acestoo high.com/.

Still, George. "Some Abnormal Physical Conditions in Children." *Lancet*, 1. (1902); 1008–1012.

Strohl, Madeleine. "Bradley's Benzedrine Studies on Children with Behavioral Disorders." *Yale Journal of Biology and Medicine* 84, no. 1 (March 2011): 27–33.

Talbot, Margaret. "Brain Gain: The Underground World of Neuroenhancing Drugs." *New Yorker*, April 27, 2009.

Thomas, Katie. "Glaxo Says It Will Stop Paying Doctors to Promote Drugs." *New York Times*, December 16, 2013.

Turkle, Sherry. *Psychoanalytic Politics: Jacques Lacan and Freud's French Revolution*. New York: Guilford Press, 1992.

Urban, Kimberly, and Wen-Jun Gao. "Performance Enhancement at the Cost of Potential Brain Plasticity: Neural Ramifications of Neurotropic Drugs in the Healthy Developing Brain." *Frontiers in Systems Neuroscience*, May 12, 2014.

Use of Methylphenidate for the Treatment of Attention Deficit Disorder. Report of the United Nations International Narcotics Control Board. New York: United Nations, 1995, 20–22.

Vallée, Manuel. "Biomedicalizing Mental Illness: The Case of Attention Deficit Disorder." *Advances in Medical Sociology* 11 (2010): 281–301.

———. "Resisting American Psychiatry: French Opposition to DSM-III, Biological Reductionism and the Pharmaceutical Ethos." *Advances in Medical Sociology* 12 (2011): 85–110.

Watson, Gretchen, and Andrea Arcona. "8 Ways to Respond to Student Drug Abuse." *Campus Safety*, April–May 2014.

Webster-Stratton, Carolyn, and Mary Hammond. "Treating Children with Early-Onset Conduct Problems: A Comparison of Child and Parent Training Interventions." *Journal of Consulting and Clinical Psychology* 65, no. 1 (1997): 93–109.

Wedge, Marilyn. "The Million Dollar Bagel: Harvard Doctor Fights Back." *Huffington Post*, January 25, 2012.

———. *Pills Are Not for Preschoolers: A Drug-Free Approach for Troubled Kids*. New York: W. W. Norton, 2012.

———. "7 Natural Ways to Help Your Child's ADHD." *Huffington Post*, September 11, 2011.

———. "Why French Kids Don't Have ADHD." *Psychology Today*, March 8, 2012.

Whitaker, Robert. *Anatomy of an Epidemic*. New York: Crown, 2010.

———. *Mad in America*. New York: Perseus, 2002.

Wellcome.ac.uk Web site. Organization, Technology Transfer Panel.

Wildeman, Christopher, et al. "The Prevalence of Confirmed Maltreatment Among US Children, 2004 to 2011." *JAMA Pediatrics* 168, no. 8 (August 2014): 706–13.

Wurtzel, Elizabeth. *Prozac Nation: Young and Depressed in America*. New York: Penguin, 1994.

"Younger Children in the Classroom Likely Over-diagnosed with ADHD: UBC Research." University of British Columbia media release, March 5, 2012. http://www.publicaffairs.ubc.ca/2012/03/05/.

Zelnik, Nathaniel, et al. "Range of Neurological Disorders on Patients with Celiac Disease." *Pediatrics* 113, no. 6 (June 6, 2004).

INDEX

· · · · · ·